easy everyday
mediterranean diet
cookbook

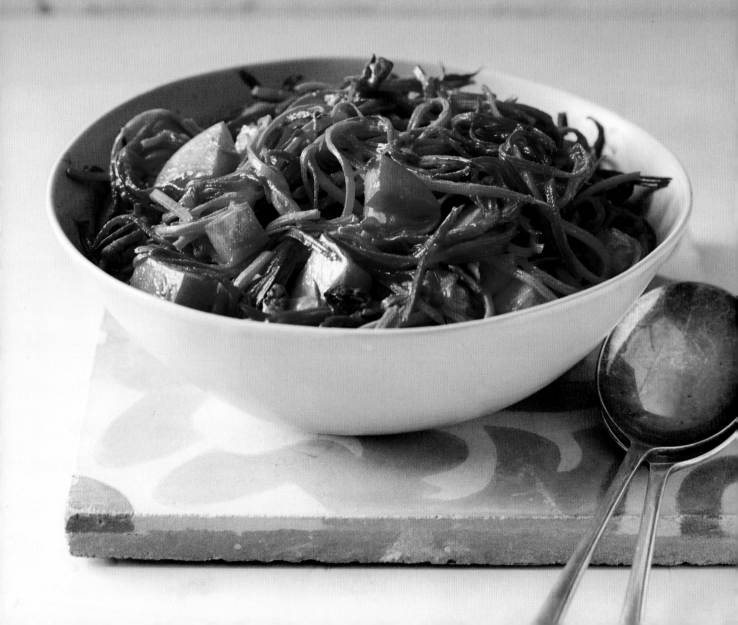

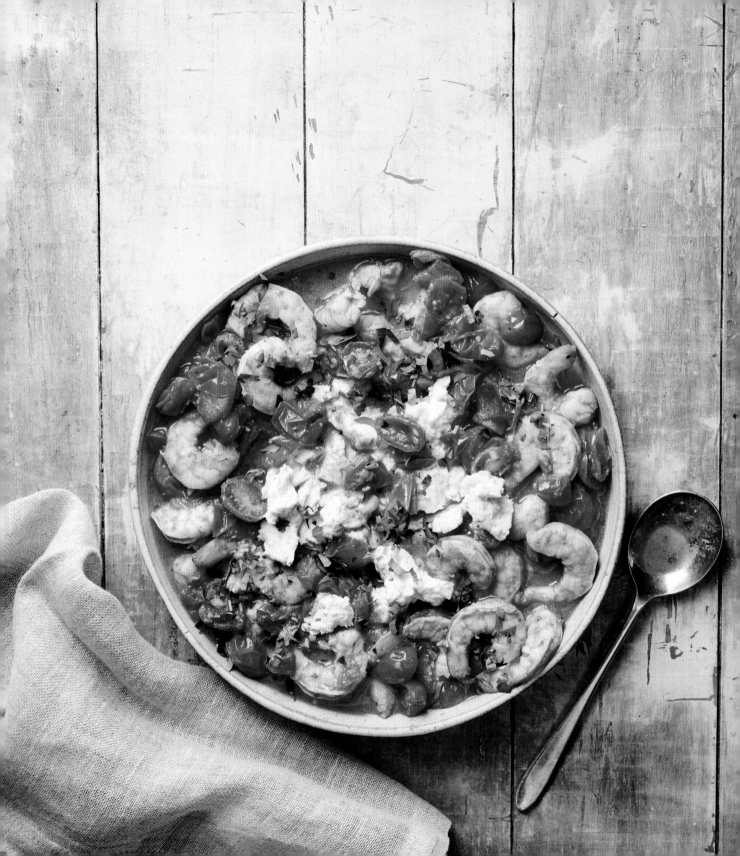

easy everyday
mediterranean diet
cookbook

125 Delicious Recipes from the Healthiest Lifestyle on the Planet

Serena Ball, MS, RD, and
Deanna Segrave-Daly, RD

Photography by Linda Xiao

Houghton Mifflin Harcourt
Boston / New York / 2020

contents

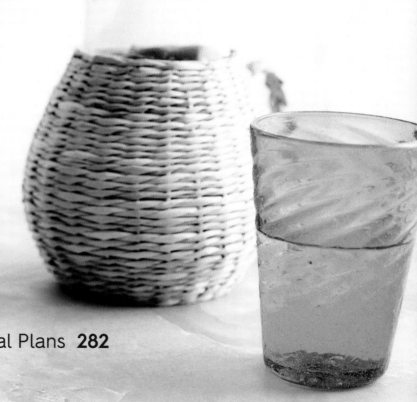

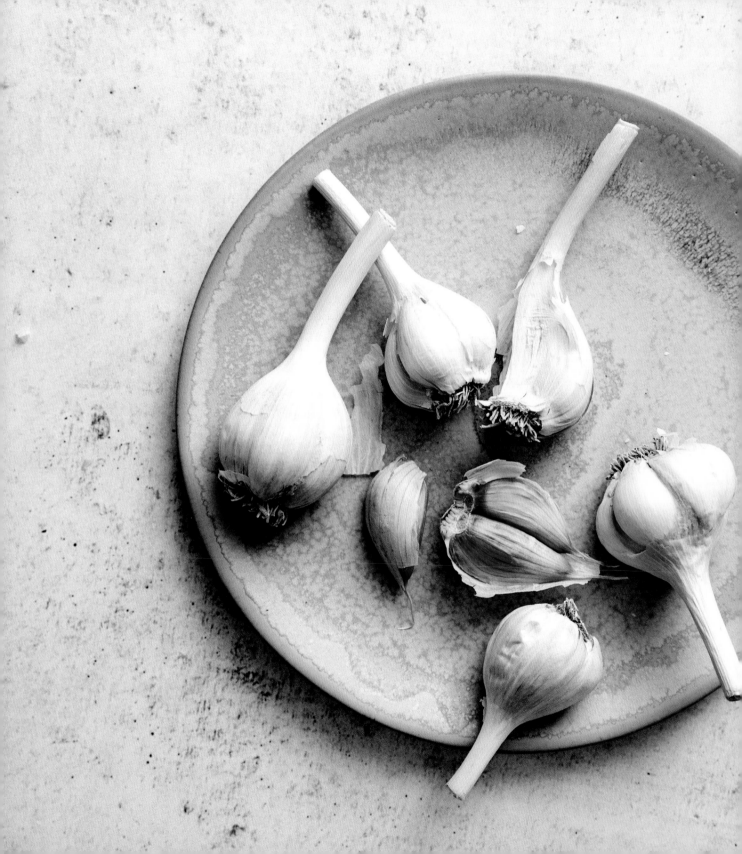

acknowledgments

A humble thank-you to Clare Pelino and Justin Schwartz, who took a chance on us, and for Stephanie Fletcher and Jacqueline Quirk, along with our HMH marketing and publicity teams, for seeing us to the finish line with this project. We are so grateful for the extraordinary talent of Linda Xiao, Kate Buckens, Tiffany Schleigh, and Maeve Sheridan for turning our recipes into visual dishes of delight. Lastly, we wouldn't be here without our loyal friends, family, readers, and diligent recipe testers—this cookbook is dedicated to all of you. xo

introduction

Quite simply, the Mediterranean Diet is a routine
of eating the delicious foods found in the regions
that border the Mediterranean Sea. Scientists have found
that eating these foods on a regular basis
can help people live longer and feel healthier.

What is the Mediterranean Diet?

The Mediterranean Diet is all about *enjoying* vibrant vegetables and fruits in season, golden lentils and creamy beans, bowls of pasta and of whole grains, tangy rich yogurt, succulent seafood, simple one-pot dishes adorned with chicken and meat and topped with piles of crisp green herbs, fresh eggs, aged cheeses, olive oil and aromatic spices, and wine on occasion.

If that's your kind of "diet" then you're in the right place!

And speaking of that word "diet," even though we are two *dietitians*, we think of this as the Mediterranean lifestyle, not a diet. That's because it's not just about what to eat (and it's certainly not about food restrictions), it's also about a rhythm of life that was rather old-fashioned but has become more top-of-mind. We're talking about (1) slowing down to enjoy our food, (2) eating with family and friends, and (3) using up food while throwing out less.

The Mediterranean countries include Italy, France, Greece, Spain, Turkey, Israel, Lebanon, Syria, Egypt, Tunisia, Morocco, Algeria, and Libya. The spices and specific dishes vary in these countries, but the food is basically the same template: plentiful vegetables, omega-3–rich fish, whole grains flavored with olive oil, spices and fresh herbs, and fermented dairy foods. These foods make up a dietary pattern that researchers have discovered is associated with many wellness benefits.

What are the health benefits?

The benefits of the Mediterranean Diet are almost as varied as the cuisines in the countries surrounding the Mediterranean Sea. They include:

Lower rates of diabetes Researchers compared a low-fat diet to a higher-fat Mediterranean Diet and found that diabetes rates were lower in people eating the Mediterranean Diet. People who have diabetes can benefit from the high fiber, good fats, quality proteins, and abundance of vegetables in the Diet.

Lower blood pressure The Mediterranean Diet is rich in extra-virgin olive oil, which may help the body remove excess cholesterol from arteries and keep blood vessels open. The healthy dietary pattern contains nutrients that can help lower blood pressure, including healthy fats, potassium, and magnesium, and is generally lower in sodium.

Less cardiovascular disease In general, eating seafood twice a week can help lower the risk of heart disease by about 36 percent. Limiting highly processed foods, added sugars, and saturated fats can help lower inflammation in the veins and arteries. Exercise, part of any Mediterranean lifestyle, helps too.

Less asthma The Mediterranean Diet is for the whole family as some studies have shown that eating this way can decrease wheezing and asthma, particularly in children. This association has even been found in babies whose mothers ate the Diet.

Reduced arthritis pain A decrease in the inflammation and pain of both osteoarthritis and rheumatoid arthritis has been associated with the Mediterranean Diet. Additionally, the Diet is rich in antioxidants, probiotics, vitamin D, and omega-3 fats, which may also decrease inflammation.

Improved brain health People eating a Mediterranean-style diet generally have a lower risk of dementia. Researchers have discovered that seafood can improve memory and sharpness in older adults. Slowing down and enjoying meals—which is less stressful—is encouraged.

Lower cancer rates Overall incidence of cancer is lower in Mediterranean countries compared to in the United States, the United Kingdom, and Scandinavian countries. Scientists on large studies looking at disease patterns have linked the Mediterranean Diet to decreased cancer incidence.

Lower mortality Researchers found that following the Mediterranean Diet reduced the risk for death from disease by 25 percent, specifically lowering the risk of coronary artery disease. And eating seafood two or three times per week reduces the risk of death from any health-related cause by 17 percent.

Increased immunity Nearly all Mediterranean Diet foods are considered "anti-inflammation" foods; eating more of them helps decrease overall chronic inflammation in the body, which researchers ultimately believe may be the root of most diseases. Since 70 percent of the immune system is located in the gut, nourishing the GI system with probiotic-rich fermented yogurt and cheeses, prebiotic-rich vegetables and beans, and antioxidant-rich whole grains, spices, fruits, and vegetables is essential.

What are the foods?

Take a look at the Mediterranean Diet Pyramid (developed originally by Oldways) to see the basic food categories and the general guidelines on what to eat on a daily basis, on a weekly basis, and in moderation.

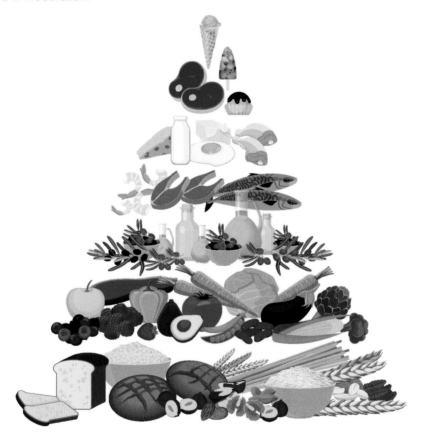

Here's how to stock your Mediterranean kitchen. See the following list of what we keep in our kitchens. You don't need everything, but keeping many ingredients on hand can lead to fewer trips to the supermarket, and fewer trips means it's easier to keep to your budget and get dinner on the table in a reasonable amount of time.

On the counter

- Fresh fruits such as apples, pears, lemons, oranges, peaches, plums, apricots, mangos, avocados
- Fresh grape tomatoes

Pantry

- Canned/jarred vegetables such as diced tomatoes, crushed tomatoes, roasted red peppers, artichokes, beets
- Canned fruit in 100 percent juice
- Canned/dried beans and lentils such as garbanzo beans; pinto beans; cannellini beans; great northern beans; brown, green, red, or yellow lentils
- Canned seafood such as salmon, tuna in olive oil, clams, sardines, shrimp
- Grains such as instant brown rice, quinoa, bulgur, farro, pearl barley, couscous
- Pasta such as white, whole grain, chickpea, lentil
- Cornmeal/tubed polenta
- Extra-virgin olive oil
- Vinegar such as rice, white wine, red wine, balsamic
- Olives such as cans or jars of black or green olives

- Capers
- Low-sodium tomato pasta sauce, tomato paste
- Low-sodium vegetable or chicken broth
- Dried fruits such as figs, prunes, apricots, raisins, dates
- Peanut butter
- Onions such as yellow, red, white
- Garlic
- Potatoes and sweet potatoes
- Butternut, acorn, and spaghetti squashes
- Beets
- Honey
- Spices (see Expand Your Mediterranean Seasoning Horizons page 15)

Refrigerator

- Nuts such as almonds, pecans, walnuts, pistachios, peanuts
- Seeds such as sesame seeds, tahini spread, ground flaxseed
- Reduced-fat (2%) milk
- Plain 2% Greek yogurt
- Aged and fresh cheeses such as ricotta, mascarpone, goat cheese, feta, mozzarella, Parmesan, Pecorino Romano, Gorgonzola
- Fresh herbs such as parsley, cilantro, basil, mint, rosemary, thyme
- Fresh vegetables such as carrots, celery, cucumbers, eggplant, leafy greens, broccoli, cauliflower, bell peppers, mushrooms, green onions
- Fresh fruits such as grapes, berries, melon, cherries
- Eggs
- Cured meat such as prosciutto, pancetta
- Chicken breasts/thighs
- 80% to 90% lean ground beef, lamb, turkey

Freezer

- Plain (unsweetened) frozen fruit such as blueberries, mango, cherries, peaches, mixed berries
- Plain frozen vegetables such as green peas, corn, spinach, green beans, cauliflower, broccoli
- Plain frozen fish fillets such as tilapia, salmon, cod
- Medium or large uncooked shrimp
- White whole-wheat flour
- Frozen gnocchi

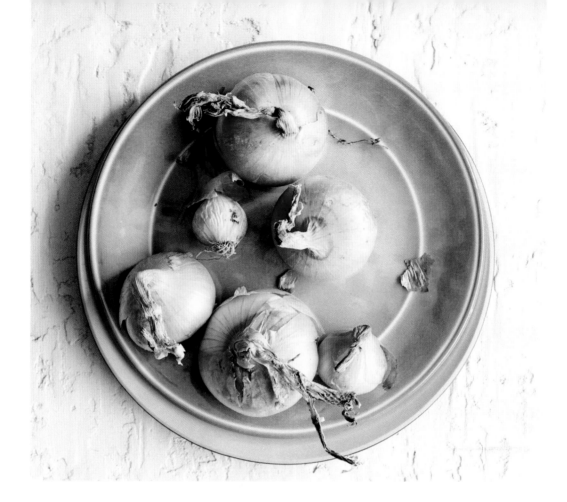

How can two dietitians, one from the Midwest and one from Philly, help you follow the Mediterranean Diet day in and day out?

We've embraced the mantra and the ingredients of the Mediterranean lifestyle for decades based on the strong nutrition research, our travels, and, more than anything, on the super-delicious yet simple cuisine.

Also, readers of our blog, TeaspoonOfSpice.com, have told us which recipes and Healthy Kitchen Hacks (kitchen shortcuts featured on our blog and also included with every single recipe in this book!) actually make their lives easier. Based on their feedback and our love for all ingredients Mediterranean, we created 125 dietitian-approved recipes for this cookbook. We then went back and asked our community for volunteer testers. And those recipe testers, who are regular home cooks from all over the US, shared their honest thoughts, which resulted in us adapting these recipes to be even more straightforward and approachable for you. You'll see the testers' actual comments and feedback throughout the book.

Five Myths about the Mediterranean Diet

One of the main reasons we wanted to write this cookbook was to encourage those hesitant to try this way of eating. If we've heard these barriers to embracing the Mediterranean way, you may have, too.

Myth: It's too expensive.

Fact: Mediterranean eating is budget friendly. Mediterranean pantry essentials are some of the most economical in the supermarket and include canned tuna, dried lentils, canned beans, canned and jarred vegetables, canned fruit, frozen fruits and vegetables, frozen seafood, whole grains like instant brown rice, boxed pasta, fresh herbs, onions and garlic, root vegetables, plain yogurt, spices, and fresh herbs. And one way to save even more on groceries is to prevent food waste (see "Simple Ways to Reduce Food Waste" on page 19).

Myth: It's time-consuming.

Fact: Many of the recipes in this book can be completed in a half hour or less. And as you start cooking more often from this book, you'll begin to see similar ingredients, cooking techniques, and recipe combinations, which will help you get more comfortable in your Mediterranean kitchen, ultimately cutting back on your prep time.

Myth: It's complicated.

Fact: A Mediterranean lifestyle can fit into a busy lifestyle. Believe us, our recipe testers were *very* vocal in reminding us when a step was fussy or tricky. We changed those steps—or removed them—with the rare exception when an extra step equaled incredible flavor. This book has several tried-and-true one-pot meals, skillet suppers, sheet-pan dinners, and even a few five-ingredient-or-less dishes. While we see (and taste) the virtues of eating seasonally, we realize that sometimes you just want to grab a quick recipe to feed your family. So, most of our dishes use produce that's available year-round and grown in many parts of the country in hothouses (like fresh herbs and grape tomatoes)—and some recipes include suggestions to use canned and frozen fruits when a particular item isn't in season.

Myth: This diet is only for people over (insert "old age" number here!).

Fact: The Mediterranean lifestyle is for the whole family! This is a diet that's yummy and beneficial to all ages. It's a diet of many superfoods, not just olive oil and wine. You're never too young to learn to eat and enjoy anti-inflammation foods. In fact, many of these recipes were taste-tested and approved by our children and our recipe testers' kids, too.

Myth: There are too many carbs.

Fact: Carbs in fruits, vegetables, whole grains, beans, and other foods are packed with benefits. People who eat more carbs live longer. And while calories from carbohydrates count, just like protein and fat calories count, carb-rich whole grains and beans are packed with important antioxidants. Fruits and vegetables supply invaluable vitamins, minerals, fiber, and phytonutrients. Mediterranean carbohydrates nourish the gut microbiome. Even plain (white) pasta can provide some of the longest-lasting energy available. The trick is not to overcook it; cook only to al dente and it will actually have a lower glycemic index (meaning the carbs will take longer to digest).

Expand Your Mediterranean
Seasoning Horizons

While many of the ingredients used in cuisines across the Mediterranean are similar, it's the herbs and spices that set them apart—a bowl of beans and rice may taste very different in Tunisia when seasoned with chili powder and coriander, than in Greece, seasoned with dill and oregano. Here are some of the combinations of spices we use in this book to help you hop on a global flavor adventure:

Greek: Dill, thyme, oregano, sage

Italian: Oregano, thyme, fennel, rosemary, crushed red pepper

Southern French: Rosemary, thyme, garlic, black pepper

Spanish: Sweet paprika, smoked paprika, garlic, parsley

Middle Eastern and Israeli: Za'atar (a mix that is often homemade; make your own with oregano, thyme, sesame seeds, and lemon zest), dried fruits, sesame seeds, parsley

North African: Turmeric, cinnamon, crushed red pepper, coriander, cilantro, sesame seeds

Turkish: Dried fruits, sesame seeds, red peppers

Across the Mediterranean: Citrus (especially lemons and oranges), olives, oregano, parsley, honey, sea salt

About our cookware: No, we don't have our own cookware line! Both of us still have many of the same pots and pans we bought in our single days or received as wedding presents two decades ago. The list below has our go-to kitchen equipment, which is used throughout this book.

- Large rimmed baking sheet (12 × 18-inch)
- Wire rack (cooling rack)
- Large skillet (12-inch). It doesn't have to be nonstick, but should have a lid (or use aluminum foil as a makeshift cover).
- Saucepan with a lid (4-quart)
- Large stockpot (8-quart)
- Cast iron skillet (10- or 12-inch)

- Baking dish—a dish is glass
- Baking pan—a pan is metal
- Microplane zester
- Meat thermometer
- Kitchen brush
- Blender or immersion blender
- Food processor or high-powered blender

About our kitchens: We are regular home cooks without fancy stoves. (In fact, some of our testers have fancier stoves!) We have gas ranges, so if you have an electric stove, some of your cooking times might be slightly longer. That's why we give ranges for most cooking times.

A note about broilers: We both have a broiler in which the heating element runs down the center of the top of the oven. If your broiler covers the entire top of your oven, watch your food extra carefully to prevent burning, as it can scorch in seconds!

Just a few disclaimers before you dive in:

We don't live in, nor are we from, the Mediterranean region. We've based this book on research, aspects of the cuisines we've enjoyed from our travels, experimenting in the kitchen, and recipes we created from ingredients we (and our recipe testers around the country) think taste delicious together.

The label "nut-free" does not mean "seed-free." We use tahini, sesame seeds, and flaxseed in several recipes that are labeled "nut-free."

This book discusses topics related to health, fitness, and nutrition. This information should not be treated as medical advice. You must not rely on the information in this book as an alternative to advice from your medical professional or healthcare provider. Please do not delay seeking medical advice, disregard medical advice, or discontinue medical treatment as a result of any information provided in this book.

Now get ready to bring some Mediterranean sunshine and scrumptious meals to your kitchen!

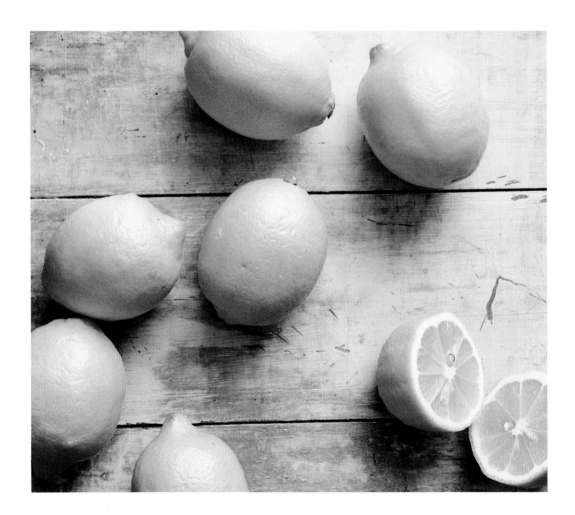

Simple Ways to Reduce Food Waste

Use up more of the ingredients you buy! Below are a few ways to waste less when cooking Mediterranean. Look for even more food-waste tips featured in Healthy Kitchen Hacks throughout the book.

Use the stems of fresh herbs. Chop up parsley and cilantro stems along with the leaves. These stems are very tender and are often sweeter than the leaves. Use in crunchy salads, blend into pesto, or chop finely and add to meatloaf and grain dishes.

Use the tough stems of leafy greens. Finely chop the stems of kale, collards, Swiss chard, and other greens. Add them first to the pan/skillet to get a head start on cooking before tossing in the leaves.

Use the leaves and stalks of veggies. There's a reason "broccoli slaw" can now be found in the produce section: the stems are crunchier and sweeter than the florets. But you can also use the trimmed stems of cauliflower, cabbage, and tender Brussels sprout stalks. Chop them finely and use as you would normally cook these veggies. (We highly recommend roasting!) And those little mini leaves on the stalks of broccoli, cauliflower, and celery, and on the top of a giant stalk of Brussels sprouts? They are tasty additions to salads or sautés.

Store your extra fresh herbs. Woody herbs like rosemary and thyme can be dried by simply laying them on the counter. Chop tender herbs like cilantro, parsley, mint, or basil, and place in ice-cube trays; then cover with orange juice, olive oil, broth, or white wine and freeze. Pop these frozen cubes into soups, tomato sauce, chili, pasta sauce, and grain dishes.

Store remaining citrus zest and juice. As they do in the Mediterranean, we use *a lot* of fresh lemons throughout this book (the acid wakes up the flavor of your food!). Before juicing a lemon, orange, or lime, always zest it right into a glass or plastic freezer container or bag (if the peel isn't used in the recipe). Extra halves of lemons, oranges, or limes can be juiced into freezer or fridge containers. After the zesting and juicing, throw spent rinds down the garbage disposal for a fresh scent; plus, the tough skin will grab trapped debris.

Roast all squash seeds. Think beyond the pumpkin and save the seeds of butternut, acorn, and spaghetti squashes. Scoop them straight into a bowl, then drizzle with olive oil and season with a pinch of salt. Place on a baking sheet and roast at 375°F for 15 to 20 minutes until toasted. And there's no need to clean those seeds before roasting—they're actually *better* with bits of squash flesh because that clingy part turns to a chewy, fruit-leather texture that's super snackable.

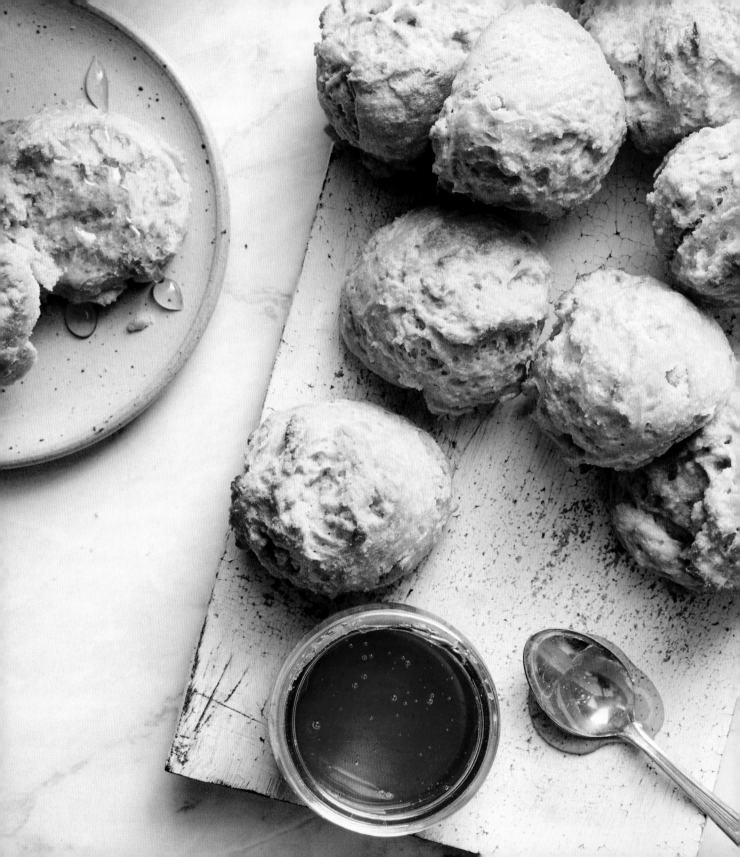

breakfast

Apple-Walnut Ricotta Toast

Egg-Free, Vegetarian		**Serves 4**	Prep time: 10 minutes	Cook time: 10 minutes

⅓ cup chopped walnuts

2 medium apples, chopped (about 2 cups)

2 teaspoons honey, divided

¼ teaspoon ground cinnamon

¾ cup whole-milk ricotta cheese

⅛ teaspoon kosher or sea salt

8 (4-inch diameter) whole-grain bread slices or 4 (8-inch) whole-grain bread slices, toasted

It's worth taking a few extra minutes in the morning to whip your ricotta for this dessert-like toast that's surprisingly packed with protein and fiber. The aroma of toasted walnuts and quick-cooking apples may also wake up your family and bring them to the kitchen!

Put the walnuts in a small skillet over medium heat. Cook, stirring occasionally, until the walnuts are lightly toasted, 4 to 6 minutes. Set aside.

While the walnuts cook, in a microwave-safe bowl, put the apples, 1 teaspoon of the honey, and the cinnamon and stir well. Microwave on high for 1 to 1½ minutes, until the apples have softened slightly. Remove the bowl and mash the apples with a fork to form a chunky apple topping. Set aside.

In a large bowl, put the ricotta, the remaining 1 tablespoon honey, and the salt. Using an electric beater or a stand mixer with the whisk attachment, whip for 1 to 2 minutes until smooth.

To assemble the toast, spread the whipped ricotta over each piece of bread with a knife or the back of a spoon. Top with the toasted walnuts and the warm apple mixture.

Healthy Kitchen Hack: Take this microwaved apple shortcut a step further to make homemade applesauce in a flash. After removing the apples from the microwave, stir in 1 tablespoon water. Return to the microwave and heat for another 1½ minutes, until the apples are very soft. Remove the bowl with oven mitts and either mash with a fork or puree in a blender. Pears also work well in this recipe to make a speedy pear sauce.

Per Serving: Calories: 342; Total Fat: 15g; Saturated Fat: 5g; Cholesterol: 24mg; Sodium: 312mg; Total Carbohydrates: 41g; Fiber: 7g; Protein: 15g

Cinnamon-Fig Granola

Dairy-Free, Gluten-Free, Egg-Free, Vegetarian	Serves 6	Prep time: 15 minutes	Cook time: 20 minutes

1 large orange

2½ cups gluten-free old-fashioned rolled oats

½ cup chopped pecans

¼ cup honey

¼ cup extra-virgin olive oil

¾ teaspoon ground cinnamon

¼ teaspoon kosher or sea salt

½ cup chopped dried figs (about 6 whole figs)

Homemade granola is fairly straightforward to make and usually has a better-for-you nutritional profile than store-bought varieties. In this version, we feature the classic Mediterranean flavors of citrus and fig that will add aroma and sweetness to your breakfast bowl, minus the crazy amount of added sugar often seen in store-bought granola.

Preheat the oven to 350°F. Line a large rimmed baking sheet with parchment paper.

With a Microplane or a citrus zester, grate the zest of the orange into a large bowl. (Save any remaining orange for another use.) Add the oats, pecans, honey, olive oil, cinnamon, and salt. Stir until all the oats are coated.

Spread the granola out on the prepared baking sheet. Bake for 18 to 20 minutes, until lightly browned, stirring halfway through the baking process. Remove from the oven and cool completely.

Mix in the chopped figs. Store in an airtight container in the pantry for up to 2 weeks.

Healthy Kitchen Hack: Of course, you can enjoy your homemade granola in a bowl with milk, mixed into a yogurt parfait, or eaten out of hand, but we have a few more out-of-the-box ideas. Toss it over roasted carrots, baked sweet potatoes, or salad greens. Mix it into pancake, waffle, or muffin batter. Sprinkle it over avocado toast or our Honey-Panzanella Fruit Bowl (page 274).

Per Serving: Calories: 338; Total Fat: 15g; Saturated Fat: 2g; Cholesterol: 0mg; Sodium: 99mg; Total Carbohydrates: 44g; Fiber: 6g; Protein: 5g

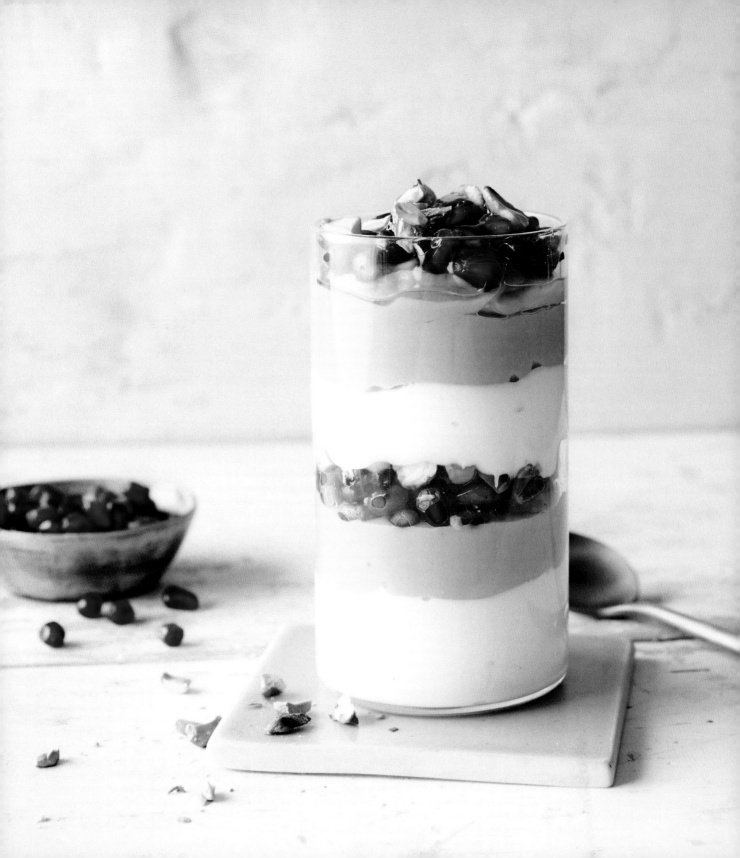

Middle Eastern Avocado-Yogurt Parfaits

Gluten-Free, Egg-Free, Vegetarian	Serves 4	Prep time: 10 minutes

2 avocados

2 tablespoons reduced-fat (2%) milk

4 teaspoons honey, divided

2 cups vanilla Greek yogurt (about 16 ounces)

½ cup pomegranate seeds (from ½ pomegranate)

¼ cup shelled pistachios

Avocados in a breakfast parfait? We say "yes"! Avocados are actually a fruit, so they are delicious when paired with honey, pomegranate seeds, and vanilla yogurt. Their creamy flesh whips up like a dream. The challenge will be for you to not eat all of the avocado layer before assembling the parfait.

Cut each avocado in half and remove the pits with a spoon. Scoop the flesh into a blender or food processor. Add the milk and 2 teaspoons of the honey. Blend until smooth.

To assemble the parfaits, spoon ¼ cup of the yogurt into each of four tall glasses. Layer with the avocado cream, divided evenly among the glasses. Top each with 1 tablespoon of pomegranate seeds and then ½ tablespoon of pistachios. Layer each with the remaining 1 cup yogurt, ¼ cup pomegranate seeds, and 2 tablespoons pistachios. Top each parfait with a drizzle of the remaining honey.

Healthy Kitchen Hack: Pomegranates are typically available during the fall and winter months but in the off season, look for frozen or freeze-dried pomegranate seeds, which are rising in popularity in grocery stores. You can also replace the seeds with chopped dried prunes, dried cherries, or dried cranberries.

Per Serving: Calories: 322; Total Fat: 16g; Saturated Fat: 3g; Cholesterol: 7mg; Sodium: 237mg; Total Carbohydrates: 39g; Fiber: 7g; Protein: 10g

Overnight Honey Breakfast Barley

Egg-Free, Vegetarian	Serves 1	Prep time: 10 minutes	Chill time: Overnight

6 ounces plain 2% Greek yogurt

⅓ cup uncooked pearl barley

1 tablespoon golden raisins or regular raisins

1 tablespoon chopped walnuts

1 teaspoon honey

1 orange

½ small mango, chopped (about ½ cup)

Move over, overnight oats! Embrace the nutty deliciousness of plumped-up barley that's been chilled in yogurt in your refrigerator. With mix-ins like golden raisins, mangoes, and orange zest, this out-of-the-bowl breakfast brings instant sunshine to your morning. For a speedier version, check out our microwave shortcut below.

In a large coffee mug or mason jar, put the yogurt, barley, raisins, walnuts, and honey.

With a Microplane or citrus zester, grate ½ teaspoon of orange zest into the mug or jar. (Save any remaining orange for another use.) Stir together and cover with plastic wrap or a lid.

Refrigerate overnight, about 8 hours for a granola-like texture or 12 hours for a cooked oatmeal texture.

Stir in the mango before serving.

Healthy Kitchen Hack: Forgot to make your overnight barley last night? No worries! Combine ⅓ cup uncooked barley and ½ cup water in a large microwave-safe bowl or quart jar and microwave on high for 1 minute. Stir and microwave for an additional 45 to 60 seconds until the barley is soft and chewy. Stir in the yogurt and the other remaining ingredients.

Per Serving: Calories: 445; Total Fat: 8g; Saturated Fat: 2g; Cholesterol: 17mg; Sodium: 65mg; Total Carbohydrates: 71g; Fiber: 8g; Protein: 24g

Cream of Polenta with Pears and Walnuts

Gluten-Free, Egg-Free, Vegetarian	Serves 6	Prep time: 5 minutes	Cook time: 20 minutes

1½ cups yellow cornmeal

2½ cups reduced-fat (2%) milk

1½ tablespoons honey

¾ teaspoon vanilla extract

¼ teaspoon ground nutmeg

¼ teaspoon kosher or sea salt

½ cup walnut pieces

2 cups chopped pears
(about 2 pears)

If you, like Deanna, have fond childhood memories of eating Cream of Wheat for breakfast or are simply looking to switch up your morning oatmeal routine, this recipe is for you! Made from cornmeal, polenta is typically used in savory dishes, but here we use milk, fresh fruit, honey, and vanilla to create a sweet and enticing way to start your day.

In a medium saucepan, whisk together the cornmeal, milk, and 1 cup warm water. Bring the mixture to a simmer over medium-high heat, whisking occasionally. Whisk in ½ cup warm water then reduce the heat to medium-low. Cook, stirring frequently, until the polenta thickens, about 15 minutes. Remove from the stove and whisk in the honey, vanilla, nutmeg, and salt.

While the polenta cooks, put the walnuts in a small dry skillet over medium heat. Cook, stirring occasionally, until the walnuts are lightly toasted, 4 to 6 minutes. Set aside.

Divide the polenta evenly among six bowls. Top each with the toasted walnuts and the chopped pears.

Healthy Kitchen Hack: To cut down on prep time, buy tubed polenta, which has already been cooked. Slice two 18-ounce tubes into rounds and microwave for 1 minute. Transfer the heated polenta to a pot and mash with a fork. Over medium heat, slowly whisk in the milk until the polenta warms. Remove the pot from the stove and follow the rest of the recipe instructions.

Per Serving: Calories: 286; Total Fat: 9g; Saturated Fat: 2g; Cholesterol: 8mg; Sodium: 611mg; Total Carbohydrates: 44g; Fiber: 5g; Protein: 8g

Prosciutto-Parsley Egg Cups

| Nut-Free, Gluten-Free | | Serves 6 | Prep time: 5 minutes | Cook time: 15 minutes |

4 ounces sliced prosciutto or 12 very thin slices deli ham

¾ cup chopped fresh parsley, plus more for garnish

12 large eggs

¼ cup reduced-fat (2%) milk

⅛ teaspoon kosher or sea salt

⅛ teaspoon black pepper

"I loved making these egg cups—they were so quick and easy! Even the cleanup was easy because the prosciutto acts as a muffin tin liner."

—Lydia from Breese, IL

These yummy egg cups make a beautiful breakfast with their orange yolks topped with bright green parsley and encased in salty prosciutto. A drizzle of milk over each cup keeps the eggs from overcooking and turning tough while baking. Make a batch of these ahead of time to have on hand for busy mornings. Wrap the cooked and cooled egg cups tightly in plastic wrap and freeze. To reheat, use the defrost setting in your microwave.

Preheat the oven to 375°F. Coat a 12-cup muffin tin with cooking spray.

Trim the prosciutto slices so they fit into each cup of the muffin tin (a small amount should hang over the edge of each muffin cup). Top the prosciutto in each cup with 1 tablespoon of the parsley. Break 1 egg into each cup. Pour 1 teaspoon of the milk over each egg and then sprinkle the salt and black pepper evenly over all the eggs.

Bake for 15 minutes or until the egg whites are just set. Remove the pan from the oven and set on a wire rack to cool for 5 minutes; the eggs will continue to cook, but the yolks will still be slightly runny and "jammy." (If you prefer more firmly set egg yolks, bake for a total of 16 to 17 minutes.)

To serve, slide a butter knife around each egg and remove gently. Garnish with extra parsley.

Healthy Kitchen Hack: Cleaning baked-on eggs out of a muffin pan is not a (Mediterranean!) breeze. To avoid using lots of elbow grease, coat the muffin cups really well with cooking spray before baking and make sure that the prosciutto covers the entire cup.

Per Serving: Calories: 188; Total Fat: 12g; Saturated Fat: 4g; Cholesterol: 376mg; Sodium: 561g; Total Carbohydrates: 2g; Fiber: 0g; Protein: 18g

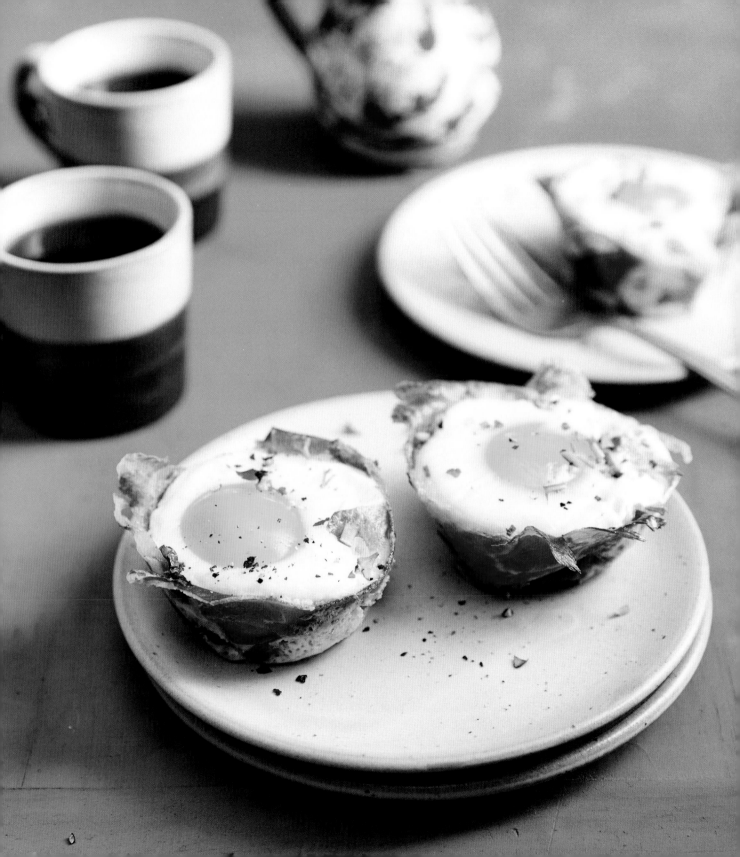

Tomato-Basil Frittata

Nut-Free, Gluten-Free, Vegetarian | **Serves 4** | Prep time: 5 minutes | Cook time: 20 minutes

5 large eggs

¼ teaspoon kosher or sea salt

1 cup fresh basil leaves, torn

2 teaspoons extra-virgin olive oil

3 medium tomatoes (or 6 to 8 Campari tomatoes), cut into ¼-inch-thick slices

½ cup shredded part-skim mozzarella cheese (about 2 ounces), divided

Tomato and basil is a classic Italian pairing that reminds us of summer all year round. Luckily, these days you can find fresh basil and decent tomatoes even in the off season at grocery stores. For the best-tasting tomatoes in the produce aisle, choose grape or Campari varieties, which are both good stand-ins for the larger fresh-from-the-garden summer tomatoes that we love to use in this layered egg dish.

Whisk the eggs and salt together in a bowl. Gently stir in the basil and set aside.

Heat a large 10- or 12-inch nonstick skillet (with a lid) over medium-low heat and pour in the olive oil. Place the tomato slices on the bottom of the pan, overlapping as necessary. Sprinkle with half of the cheese. Pour the egg mixture over the top. Sprinkle with the remaining cheese. Cover and cook until the eggs are just set, 15 to 18 minutes. Do not overcook, as the eggs will continue to cook after the skillet is removed from the heat. Serve warm or at room temperature.

Healthy Kitchen Hack: Basil leaves are very fragile. They turn brown quickly after slicing because the knife blade bruises the leaf edges. For a gentler approach, tear the basil leaves. High heat can also turn basil brown; so only add the herb to cool or room-temperature dishes—or heat slowly as we do with our frittata here.

Per Serving: Calories: 178; Total Fat: 11g; Saturated Fat: 4g; Cholesterol: 242mg; Sodium: 313mg; Total Carbohydrates: 7g; Fiber: 2g; Protein: 13g

Spanish Potato Tortilla

Dairy-Free, Nut-Free, Gluten-Free, Vegetarian	Serves 6	Prep time: 5 minutes	Cook time: 15 minutes

7 large eggs

¼ teaspoon kosher or sea salt

2 tablespoons extra-virgin olive oil

4½ cups frozen cubed potatoes with onions and peppers (from a 28-ounce package)

½ cup roasted red peppers from a jar or Roasted Red Peppers (page 44), sliced into strips

"I loved how easy this was to make and serve—right from the skillet. It was delicious!"

—Catherine from Havertown, PA

A Spanish tortilla is actually a traditional Spanish omelet made with plenty of olive oil, potatoes, eggs, and often onions. It's the simplicity of this dish that makes it so delicious, not to mention a great breakfast choice for a busy morning. Imagine you're in sunny Spain as you enjoy this hearty morning meal either hot from the pan or at room temperature.

Place the top oven rack about 4 inches below the broiler heating element. Preheat the broiler to high.

In a medium bowl, whisk the eggs and salt together and set aside.

Put a 12-inch oven-safe nonstick skillet over medium heat and pour in the oil. Sprinkle the frozen potatoes over the oil. Cook, stirring occasionally to break apart any frozen clumps of potatoes, for 8 minutes. Then continue to cook, but without stirring so some potatoes turn golden, for 4 more minutes. Pour the eggs over the potatoes and stir occasionally until the eggs begin to set but are not yet firm, 2 to 3 minutes. Place the skillet under the broiler and broil for 2 to 3 minutes until the eggs are set and just beginning to turn golden brown.

Using oven mitts, remove the hot skillet from the oven. Slide a heatproof silicone scraper around the edges and under the tortilla to loosen it from the skillet. To flip out the tortilla, use oven mitts to hold the skillet handle with one hand and then invert the tortilla onto a serving plate held beneath the skillet. Top the tortilla with the roasted red peppers and then cut it into six wedges.

Healthy Kitchen Hack: For most of our recipes, we use a regular skillet. However, for egg dishes, a nonstick skillet helps make cleanup a breeze. If you don't have one for this tortilla, you can still make it as directed, but serve it directly from the skillet instead of inverting it onto a serving plate.

Per Serving: Calories: 176; Total Fat: 10g; Saturated Fat: 3g; Cholesterol: 217mg; Sodium: 348mg; Total Carbohydrates: 13g; Fiber: 2g; Protein: 8g

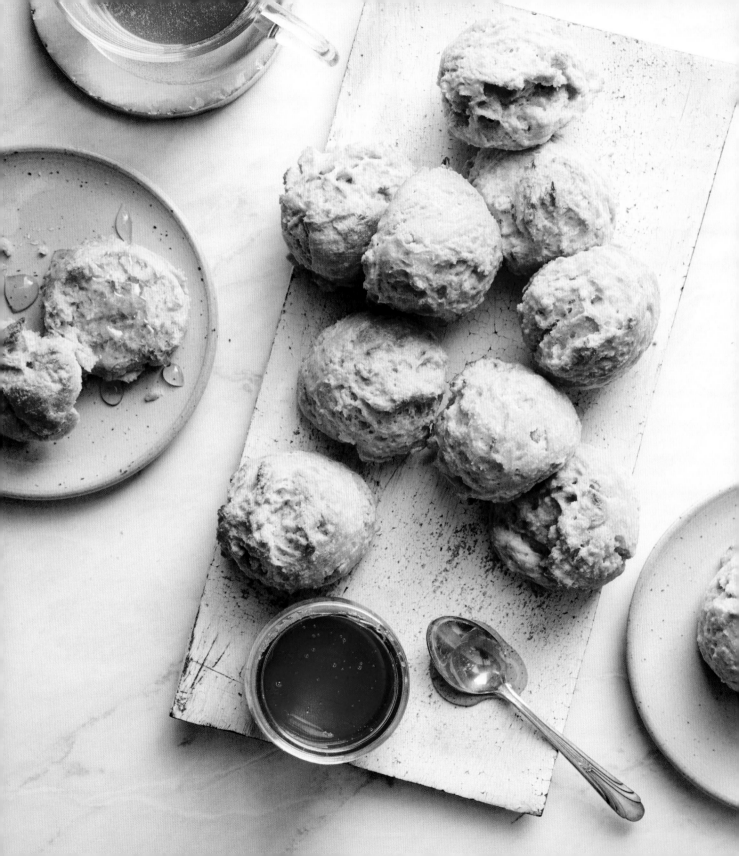

Breakfast Biscuits

Nut-Free, Egg-Free, Vegetarian	Serves 12	Prep time: 10 minutes	Cook time: 10 minutes

2 cups white
whole-wheat flour

1 tablespoon baking powder

½ teaspoon kosher or sea salt

⅓ cup extra-virgin olive oil

¾ cup plain 2% Greek yogurt
(6 ounces)

¼ cup plus 2 tablespoons
reduced-fat (2%) milk,
divided

Optional breakfast sandwich
fillings: aged salami, cheese,
Roasted Red Peppers
(page 44), pear slices, salad
greens

"These biscuits have
a great texture and
are surprisingly light
for a whole-wheat
biscuit. And I feel
good about using
whole-wheat flour
for extra nutrition
for my kids."

—Angela from Denison, IA

These baking powder biscuits are light and feathery, but sturdy enough to hold a host of sandwich fillings stacked inside for a grab-and-go breakfast. They are also enriched with tangy Greek yogurt—the Mediterranean version of buttermilk—and buttery extra-virgin olive oil. Your heart will start the day happy.

Preheat the oven to 450°F. Line a large rimmed baking sheet with parchment paper.

In a large bowl, whisk together the flour, baking powder, and salt. With a fork, stir in the olive oil until the dough is crumbly. Add the yogurt and ¼ cup of the milk and stir just until all the dry ingredients are incorporated.

With a 2-inch cookie scoop (or a ¼-cup measuring cup), scoop out 12 equal portions of dough onto the lined baking sheet. Brush the biscuit tops with the remaining milk.

Bake for 9 to 11 minutes, until the biscuits just begin to turn slightly golden. Do not overbake. Cut the biscuits in half horizontally and serve plain or with honey or fill with optional breakfast sandwich ingredients.

Healthy Kitchen Hack: Make these the night before and cool overnight on a wire rack covered with a clean kitchen towel. In the morning, warm the biscuits under the broiler for no more than 1 minute (watch carefully). Cut the biscuits in half and fill with your favorite breakfast sandwich ingredients. To freeze, wrap each biscuit individually in plastic wrap or parchment paper. Place in a plastic zip-top bag and freeze for up to 6 months. To reheat, place frozen biscuits on a lined baking sheet. Bake at 350°F for 12 to 15 minutes, until hot.

Per Serving (2 plain biscuits): Calories: 275; Total Fat: 14g; Saturated Fat: 3g; Cholesterol: 5mg; Sodium: 183mg; Total Carbohydrates: 33g; Fiber: 4g; Protein: 9g

Peanut Butter–Apricot Breakfast Oat Bars

| Gluten-Free, Vegetarian | Serves 9 | Prep time: 10 minutes | Cook time: 30 minutes |

3 cups gluten-free old-fashioned rolled oats

2 teaspoons baking powder

2 teaspoons ground cinnamon

¼ teaspoon kosher or sea salt

⅔ cup reduced-fat (2%) milk

½ cup plain 2% Greek yogurt

½ cup applesauce

¼ cup plus 1 tablespoon peanut butter, divided

4 tablespoons honey, divided

3 tablespoons extra-virgin olive oil

2 large eggs

1 teaspoon vanilla extract

¾ cup dried apricots, chopped (about 20 apricots)

Deanna has been making a version of this baked oatmeal for her family for years. Here, she gives it a Mediterranean twist by using olive oil instead of canola oil, substituting honey for the brown sugar, and adding dried apricots for sweetness, color, and nutrients. Feel free to swap in your favorite dried fruit—such as raisins, cranberries, or figs—or even fresh or frozen fruit, such as blueberries, strawberries, or cherries.

Preheat the oven to 350°F. Coat an 8-inch square baking pan with cooking spray.

Into a large bowl, measure the oats, baking powder, cinnamon, and salt. Mix together and set aside.

In another large bowl, put the milk, yogurt, applesauce, 3 tablespoons of the peanut butter, 3 tablespoons of the honey, the olive oil, eggs, and vanilla and mix together. Pour the wet ingredients into the dry ingredients and mix until just incorporated. Add the dried apricots and carefully mix in. Pour the batter into the prepared baking pan and spread evenly. Bake for 30 minutes until golden brown on top and the middle tests clean with a toothpick. Cool slightly.

In a small bowl, put the remaining 2 tablespoons peanut butter and 1 tablespoon honey. Whisk together. If too thick to spread, whisk in a teaspoon of water. Thinly spread over the baked oatmeal and then cut into 9 bars. (Note: You can make these ahead of time without the spread. Cut and seal the bars in the pan in plastic wrap. Store in the refrigerator for up to 4 days. Let them come to room temperature and spread with the peanut butter–honey topping before serving.)

continued

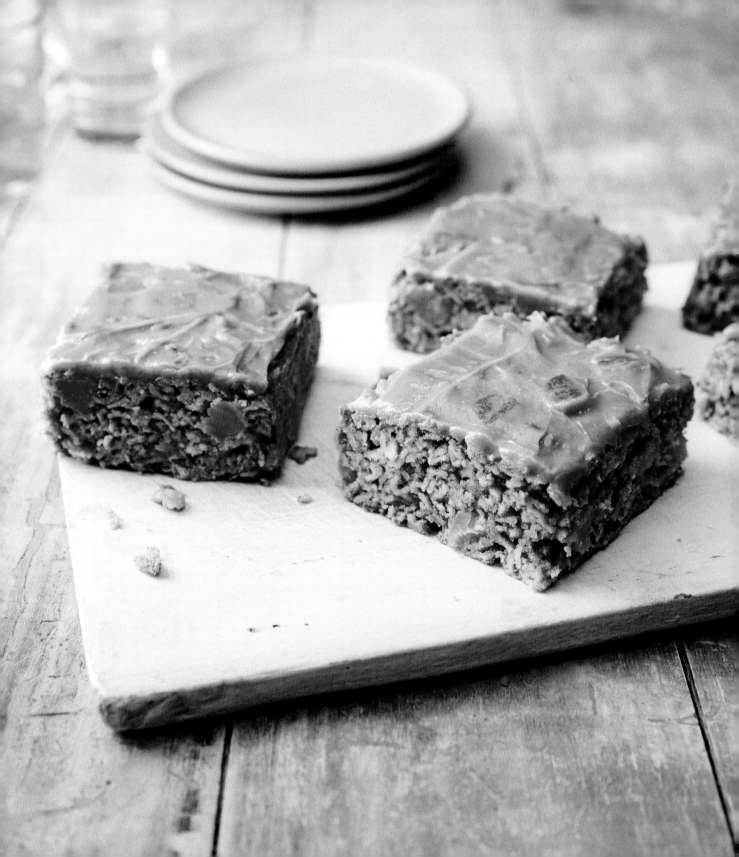

Peanut Butter–Apricot Breakfast Oat Bars (continued)

Healthy Kitchen Hack: Turn this recipe into a family-size serving of no-cook overnight oats. Omit the baking powder, olive oil, and eggs. Mix all the remaining ingredients together in a large bowl and cover. Let sit in the refrigerator overnight and by morning, the oats will have plumped up and taken on the flavors of the other ingredients.

Per Serving: Calories: 292; Total Fat: 11g; Saturated Fat: 3g; Cholesterol: 44mg; Sodium: 129mg; Total Carbohydrates: 40g; Fiber: 4g; Protein: 9g

"These came out perfectly baked! I had them at night but think they'd be great for breakfast to get you through the morning."

—Ian from Chester Springs, PA

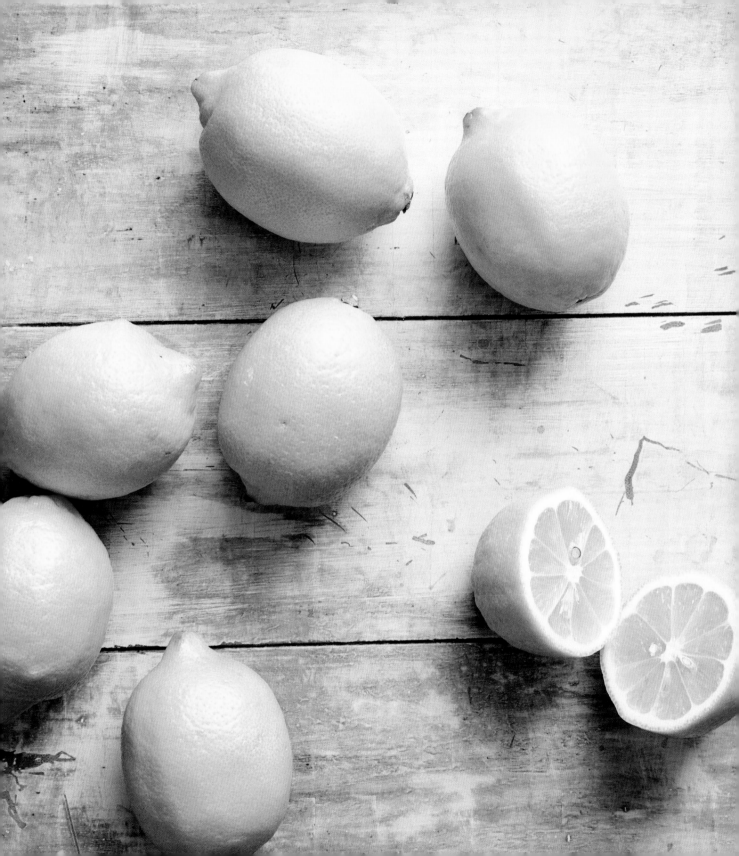

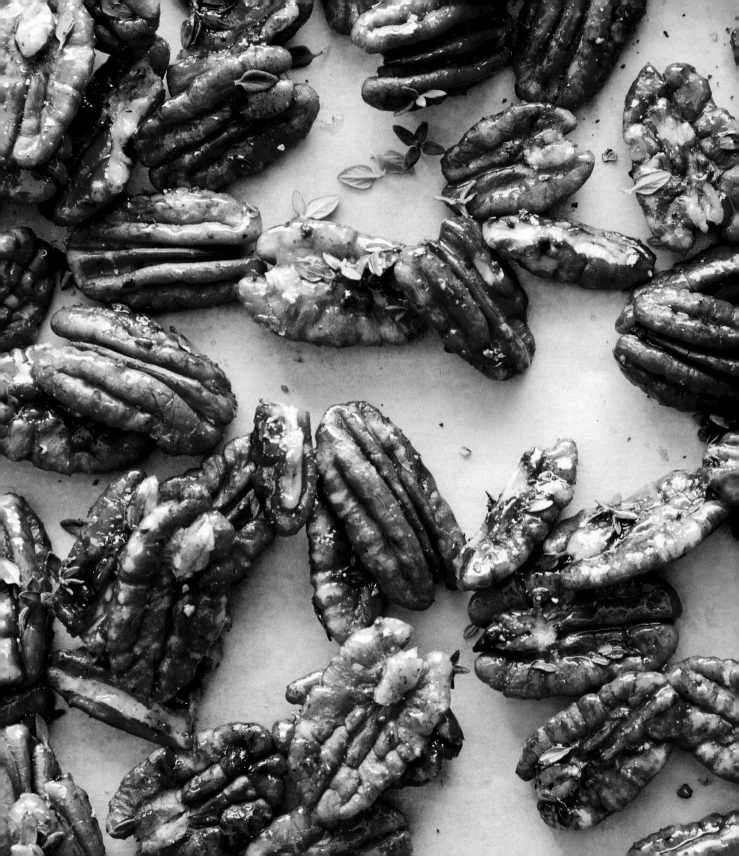

small plates and snacks

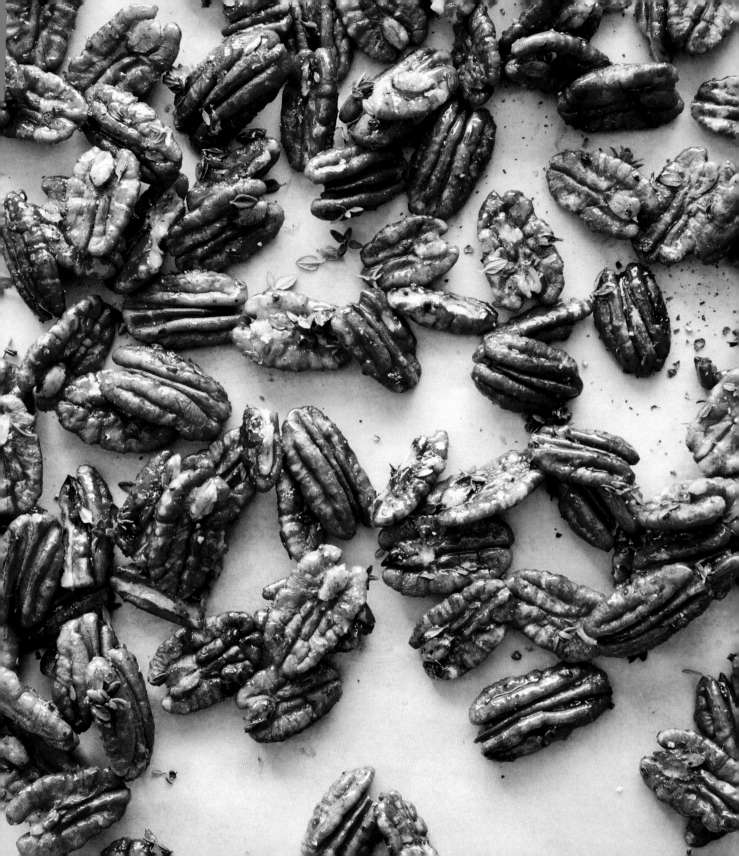

Honey-Roasted Pecans with Thyme

Dairy-Free, Gluten-Free, Egg-Free, Vegetarian	Serves 8	Prep time: 5 minutes	Cook time: 10 minutes

1¼ cups pecan halves

2 teaspoons chopped fresh thyme leaves

¼ teaspoon black pepper

¼ teaspoon kosher or sea salt

1 tablespoon honey

Warning: These sweet and peppery pecans are so yummy, you may be munching on them before they cool down. They can be whipped up in less than 15 minutes, so Deanna likes to transfer the cooled pecans to a mason jar and give them as a last-minute gift. Mix them into breakfast cereals like our Cream of Polenta with Pears and Walnuts (page 27) or toss them over fresh greens like our Arugula with Apricot Balsamic Vinaigrette (page 62).

Lay a piece of parchment paper on a baking sheet or heatproof surface.

Heat a large skillet over medium heat and add the pecans, thyme, pepper, and salt. Stir frequently until the nuts are warm, about 2 minutes.

Add the honey and cook, stirring frequently, until the nuts are completely coated and start to smell toasted, 3 to 4 minutes.

Remove the skillet from the heat and spread the nuts on the parchment paper. Cool completely (the nuts will still be somewhat sticky).

Store in an airtight container.

Healthy Kitchen Hack: For an instant breakfast muesli cereal, mix together 2 tablespoons of the Honey Roasted Pecans with ½ cup old-fashioned oats and 2 tablespoons of your favorite chopped dried fruit. Enjoy in a bowl with milk or mixed into yogurt.

Per Serving: Calories: 154; Total Fat: 15g; Saturated Fat: 1g; Cholesterol: 0mg; Sodium: 80mg; Total Carbohydrates: 6g; Fiber: 2g; Protein: 2g

Olive Oil–Yogurt Spread

Nut-Free, Gluten-Free, Egg-Free, Vegetarian	Serves 6	Prep time: 5 minutes

½ cup plain 2% Greek yogurt (4 ounces)

1 tablespoon extra-virgin olive oil

¼ teaspoon kosher or sea salt

¼ teaspoon za'atar (optional)

During her visit to Israel, Deanna discovered that many savory, spicy, or meaty entrées and side dishes were paired with plain unsweetened yogurt. This Olive Oil–Yogurt Spread is an inspiration from that trip. It's extremely versatile—whisk in any herb or spice of your choice and serve it with raw vegetables as a dip. Or mix in ⅓ cup chopped olives with a few tablespoons of olive brine from the jar and serve this yogurt spread over beef, chicken, or fish. Think of it as your new mayonnaise!

Into a large bowl, measure the yogurt, olive oil, salt, and za'atar (if using). Mix all the ingredients together with a whisk until evenly distributed. Use immediately or store in the refrigerator in a well-sealed container for up to 1 week.

Healthy Kitchen Hack: Za'atar is a staple seasoning blend in Middle Eastern cuisine and deserves a place in your pantry (as it's now available in mainstream grocery stores). "Za'atar" is also the word for a type of oregano, but the za'atar commonly sold is a mix of herbs and spices typically made up of dried thyme, dried oregano, toasted sesame seeds, and ground sumac (a tangy, lemon-flavored spice). If you don't have za'atar on hand, you can swap in an Italian seasoning blend.

Per Serving: Calories: 34; Total Fat: 3g; Saturated Fat: 1g; Cholesterol: 2mg; Sodium: 410mg; Total Carbohydrates: 1g; Fiber: 0g; Protein: 2g

Blackberry-Almond Energy Bites

Dairy-Free, Gluten-Free, Egg-Free, Vegetarian	Serves 8	Prep time: 15 minutes

¾ cup frozen blackberries

½ cup gluten-free rolled oats (old-fashioned or quick-cooking)

½ chopped almonds

¼ cup ground flaxseed

¼ teaspoon kosher or sea salt

½ cup peanut butter

2 tablespoons honey

1 teaspoon vanilla extract

"My two boys like these even better than store-bought granola bars. And I liked how quickly they came together with what I already had in the pantry. I made them with frozen cherries—yum!"

—April from Pendleton, OR

Almond trees thrive in the Mediterranean climate, so it is not surprising that we use almonds a lot throughout this cookbook. These sweet, nutrient-rich snacks are a favorite among adults and kids alike. By using frozen fruit, you don't have to chill the batter before the shaping process, which is usually the case when making no-bake nut butter bites. You (or the kids) can whip these up in no time.

Let the frozen blackberries thaw on the counter for 5 minutes, then place on a cutting board. Chop the berries with a large knife using a rocking motion, with one hand on the knife handle and the palm of your other hand near the tip of the knife.

In a large bowl, whisk together the oats, almonds, flaxseed, and salt. Add the chopped blackberries, peanut butter, honey, and vanilla. Using a wooden spoon or a fork, mix well until a dough is formed. (If the dough is too wet, add another 1 to 2 tablespoons oats.)

Lightly wet your hands to keep the dough from sticking. To assemble each bite, scoop 1½ tablespoons of dough into your palm and roll into a ball. Serve immediately or store in a sealed container in the refrigerator for up to a week or in the freezer for up to 3 months.

Healthy Kitchen Hack: These treats are infinitely adaptable. Each ingredient can be swapped out for another. Instead of blackberries, use chopped slightly thawed frozen cherries, strawberries, or blueberries. Try different nuts for almonds or a different nut butter for the peanut butter. Swap in chia seeds for ground flaxseed. Add almond extract instead of vanilla—just cut the amount to ¼ teaspoon.

Per Serving (2 bites): Calories: 212, Total Fat: 14g; Saturated Fat: 2g; Cholesterol: 0mg; Sodium: 130mg; Total Carbohydrates: 17g; Fiber: 4g; Protein: 7g

Roasted Red Peppers

Dairy-Free, Nut-Free, Gluten-Free, Egg-Free, Vegan	Serves 4	Prep time: 5 minutes	Cook time: 15 minutes

3 large or 4 medium red bell peppers

While jarred roasted peppers are a staple ingredient in our pantries, we also find that it's fairly straightforward—and empowering—to make your own using your broiler. We slice the peppers in a way that allows each piece to roast quickly, versus the more common method of roasting the entire pepper, which can be time-consuming and messy. Serve them as a side dish or as an addition to a cheese plate, or try them tossed into salads, mixed into grain dishes, spooned over chicken, or as a part of our Htipiti (Whipped Feta and Red Pepper Spread, page 56) or Rosemary-Roasted Pork and Provolone Sandwiches (page 112).

Place the top oven rack to about 4 inches below the broiler. Preheat the broiler to high. Line a large rimmed baking sheet with aluminum foil with an extra inch overlapping each end.

On a cutting board, place a pepper on its side. Slice off the top, about ½ inch from the stem. Scrape the seeds and the white membrane out of the top with your knife. Carefully cut around the green stem and remove, resulting in a circle of flesh with a small round opening in the middle. Place the circle on the prepared baking sheet, skin-side up. Discard the stem.

Cut the body of the pepper in half lengthwise. Scrape out any remaining seeds and membrane with your knife. Place both pieces skin-side up on the baking sheet and press down until each piece lies flat. Repeat with the remaining peppers.

continued

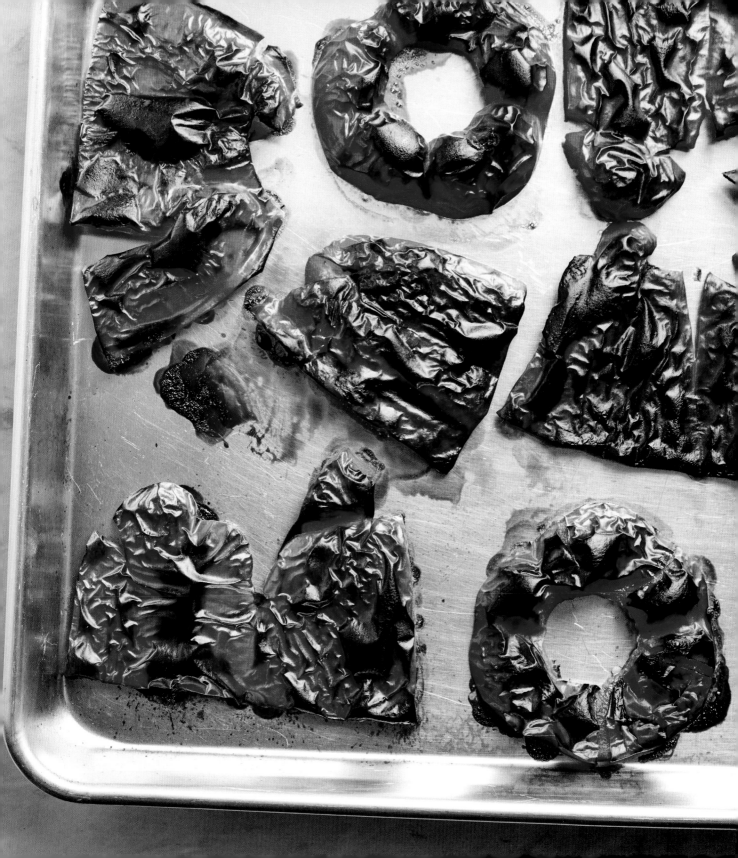

Roasted Red Peppers (continued)

Put the peppers under the broiler and broil until the skins have blackened and blistered, 10 to 12 minutes. Remove from the oven and carefully fold the foil loosely into a tent, enclosing the peppers so they continue to steam. Let the tented peppers cool on a wire rack for 10 minutes or until they are cool enough to handle.

Peel off the pepper skins with your hands and discard or add to your compost bin. Cut the peppers into strips and store in a sealed container in the refrigerator for up to 1 week.

Healthy Kitchen Hack: Puree your roasted peppers in a blender. Mix ½ to ¾ cup of the pureed peppers into tomato-based soups, chilis like our Mediterranean Lentil Chili (page 96), and pasta or pizza sauces to add superior smoky and sweet flavor.

Per Serving: Calories: 38; Total Fat: 0g; Saturated Fat: 0g; Cholesterol: 0mg; Sodium: 5mg; Total Carbohydrates: 7g; Fiber: 3g; Protein: 1g

"I love how easy these were to make compared to the traditional way of holding peppers with tongs and roasting over a flame on a stove. These are SO much better than store-bought!"

—Anne from Cherry Hill, NJ

Garlicky White Bean Tapas

Dairy-Free, Nut-Free, Gluten-Free, Egg-Free, Vegan	Serves 6	Prep time: 5 minutes	Cook time: 10 minutes

2 tablespoons extra-virgin olive oil

2 garlic cloves, minced

1 tablespoon dried oregano

¼ teaspoon crushed red pepper

¼ teaspoon kosher or sea salt

¼ teaspoon black pepper

1 (15-ounce) can cannellini beans, drained and rinsed

1 medium lemon, cut in half

Cut vegetables and toasted whole-wheat pita bread, cut into wedges, for serving (optional)

If you want an upgrade to that same old bean dip, add this dish to your list of go-to apps. Here, we mash some of the creamy cannellinis to create a super-scoopable texture that is a perfect match with raw veggies, flatbread, pita, or focaccia. The spices are warmed in olive oil to release their essence, making the oil extra aromatic and flavorful. Experiment with the different herb and spice combos we feature in our Healthy Kitchen Hack to find your favorite variation.

Heat a medium saucepan over medium-low heat and add the olive oil, garlic, oregano, crushed red pepper, salt, and black pepper. Cook, stirring occasionally, for 5 minutes.

Put the beans into a medium bowl and, using a fork or potato masher, mash about half of them. Add all the beans to the warm oil and cook, stirring occasionally, until warmed through, 2 to 3 minutes.

Squeeze 2 tablespoons of lemon juice over the warm beans and stir. (Save any remaining lemon for another use.) Transfer the bean dip to a flat serving dish with low sides. Serve with vegetables and pita bread if desired.

Healthy Kitchen Hack: Adapt this dip to flavor combinations from around the Mediterranean. For some Israeli flair, add ¼ teaspoon each of za'atar and sesame seeds. Feeling Greek love? Add 1 tablespoon each of chopped fresh dill and crumbled feta cheese. Or try a North African spice mix of ½ teaspoon ground cumin, ¼ teaspoon ground cinnamon, and ¼ teaspoon ground cardamom.

Per Serving (dip only): Calories: 99; Total Fat: 5g; Saturated Fat: 1g; Cholesterol: 0mg; Sodium: 151mg; Total Carbohydrates: 12g; Fiber: 4g; Protein: 4g

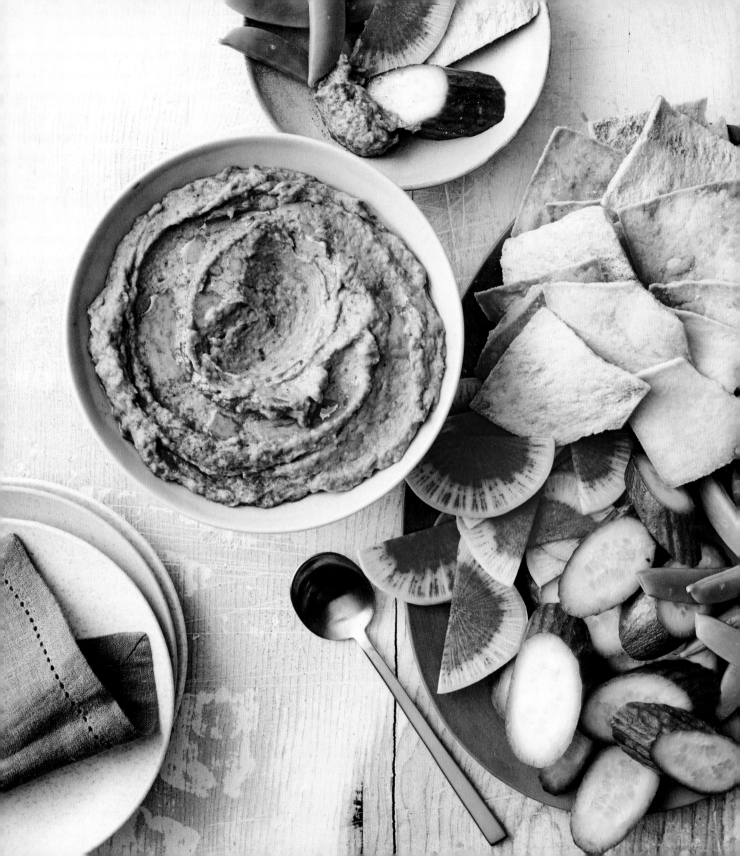

Smoky Baba Ghanoush Dip

Dairy-Free, Nut-Free, Gluten-Free, Egg-Free, Vegan	Serves 12	Prep time: 5 minutes	Cook time: 15 minutes

2 globe eggplants (about 2 pounds)

1 medium lemon, cut in half

2 tablespoons tahini or peanut butter (see Healthy Kitchen Hack below)

1 tablespoon plus 1 teaspoon extra-virgin olive oil, divided

2 garlic cloves, minced

1 teaspoon smoked paprika, divided

¼ teaspoon kosher or sea salt

Eggplant is king throughout Mediterranean cuisine, and we've made this iconic eggplant spread even easier to whip up by taking advantage of the broiler, which quickly softens the vegetable. When we serve this as a dip with pita and raw veggies, we sprinkle chopped fresh parsley, cilantro, and sesame seeds on top. It's also yummy as a sandwich spread or a replacement for tomato sauce when making pizza at home.

Place an oven rack about 4 inches under the broiler heat source. Preheat the broiler to high. Coat a large rimmed baking sheet with cooking spray.

Cut the stems off of the eggplants. Cut each eggplant lengthwise into 4 to 6 slabs (about ½ inch thick) and then place them onto the prepared baking sheet. Broil in (turning the slabs halfway through with tongs) for 10 to 12 minutes, until the eggplant flesh softens. Remove the baking sheet from the oven and place it on a wire rack to cool for 5 minutes.

Squeeze 1 tablespoon of lemon juice into a food processor or blender. (Save any remaining lemon for another use.) Add half of the eggplant slabs, the tahini, 1 tablespoon of the olive oil, the garlic, ¾ teaspoon of the smoked paprika, and the salt. Process until smooth and then add the remaining eggplant. Continue to process until smooth. (If the baba ghanoush is too thick, add a few teaspoons of water.) Put in a serving bowl, drizzle with the remaining 1 teaspoon olive oil and sprinkle with the remaining ¼ teaspoon smoked paprika, then serve, or store in the refrigerator in a well-sealed container for up to 1 week.

continued

Healthy Kitchen Hack: Tahini is sesame paste and is an Eastern Mediterranean staple ingredient. It is becoming easier to find in grocery stores (usually stocked in the international or natural foods aisle), but if you don't have it on hand, peanut butter is a terrific swap because it mimics the nutty flavor and texture of the sesame seed paste. We often use peanut butter to **make a shortcut hummus** by combining 2 tablespoons peanut butter with one 15-ounce can of chickpeas (drained, but save the liquid!), 2 tablespoons extra-virgin olive oil, and ¼ teaspoon kosher or sea salt in a food processor or a blender. Add 2 tablespoons of the reserved chickpea liquid and blend. If you like a thinner hummus, add another tablespoon of the chickpea liquid. We use this hummus recipe in our Spiced Carrot Hummus Bowls (page 207) and Flat Iron Steak, Onions, and Tomatoes over Hummus (page 228).

Per Serving: Calories: 51; Total Fat: 3g; Saturated Fat: 1g; Cholesterol: 0 mg; Sodium: 51mg; Total Carbohydrates: 7g; Fiber: 3g; Protein: 2g

"This was my first time cooking eggplant. The recipe was easy to follow, and I liked the consistency with a hint of lemon flavor."

—Liz from Collegeville, PA

Spicy Sweet Quick Pickles

Dairy-Free, Nut-Free, Gluten-Free, Egg-Free, Vegan	Serves 6	Prep time: 5 minutes	Cook time: 10 minutes

4 cups pickle-size pieces raw vegetables (see Healthy Kitchen Hack below), such as cucumbers, carrots, radishes, cauliflower, baby zucchini, baby eggplant, green beans, mini bell peppers, hot peppers, or any combination

1½ cups rice vinegar or white wine vinegar

2 tablespoons sugar

1½ tablespoons kosher or sea salt

1 knob (about 1 inch square) fresh ginger, peeled and halved

⅛ teaspoon crushed red pepper

Did you know you can make homemade pickles in minutes with almost any fresh vegetable? Small dishes of pickled vegetables are common staples on Mediterranean tables from Turkey to North Africa. Here we use fresh ginger for its natural sweetness and peppery flavor, which is popular in Middle Eastern–style pickles, but you could swap in dill for a Greek twist. Add them to our Roasted Grapes Cheese Plate (page 53) or top them on any sandwich like our Falafel Wraps (page 120) or Turkey Shawarma (page 259).

Place the vegetables in two pint-size mason jars or a large heatproof glass bowl.

In a medium saucepan, put 1½ cups water and the vinegar, sugar, salt, ginger, and crushed red pepper, stirring together. Heat the liquid over medium-high heat until it boils, stirring occasionally. Remove the pan from the stove. If using mason jars, use a spoon to remove both halves of the ginger and add one to each jar. Carefully pour the hot brine over the vegetables. Cover the mason jars with lids or the bowl with plastic wrap.

Refrigerate the pickles for 1 to 3 days before serving for the desired degree of flavor. Eat within 2 weeks.

Healthy Kitchen Hack: For "pickle-size" pieces of vegetables, think about what shape you can easily fish out of a mason jar. Slice cucumbers, carrots, and radishes into ¼-inch-thick coins. Cut cauliflower, baby zucchini, and baby eggplant into 1-inch pieces. Keep green beans, mini bell peppers, and hot peppers whole.

Per Serving: Calories: 31; Total Fat: 0g; Saturated Fat: 0g; Cholesterol: 0mg; Sodium: 269mg; Total Carbohydrates: 7g; Fiber: 1g; Protein: 1g

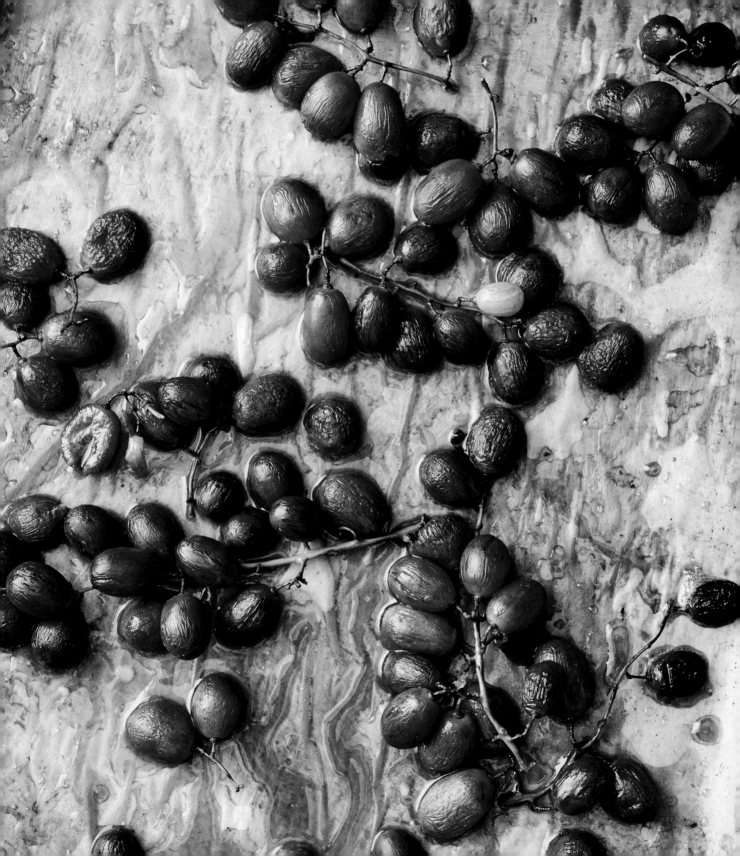

Roasted Grapes Cheese Plate

Egg-Free, Vegetarian	Serves 6	Prep time: 10 minutes	Cook time: 20 minutes

2 pounds seedless grapes, any variety or color

1 tablespoon extra-virgin olive oil

¾ cup nuts such as almonds, peanuts, pecans, pistachios, or walnuts

3 cups chopped (bite-size pieces) raw vegetables such as bell peppers, carrots, cauliflower, celery, or cucumbers

1 cup chopped (bite-size pieces) aged cheese such as Asiago, cheddar, feta, halloumi, or Manchego (about 4 ounces)

18 whole-grain crackers

Make your next cheese platter a game changer with these irresistible roasted grapes. The first time Deanna made a batch, she couldn't believe how easy they were—you don't even need to remove the stems before popping them into the oven. Each bite is like a burst of warm grape jelly—a wonderful flavor pairing to the cheeses, nuts, and grains you'll find on a classic Mediterranean snacking platter. Use the leftover grapes to top oatmeal, salads, grain dishes, or desserts.

Preheat the oven to 425°F. Line a large rimmed baking sheet with parchment paper. Spread the grapes on the baking sheet, keeping them on the stems. Using kitchen shears, snip the grapes into bunches to ensure that each grape is touching the parchment. Brush with the olive oil.

Bake for 20 minutes, until the grapes appear shrunken. Remove the pan from the oven and cool on a wire rack. Use half of the grapes for the cheese plate and store the remaining grapes in a sealed container in the refrigerator for up to a week.

Place the nuts in small bowls.

On a serving platter or large wooden board, arrange the roasted grapes, vegetables, cheeses, nuts, and crackers.

Healthy Kitchen Hack: Use this same roasting method with other fruit. We love roasting orange slices, as the rinds caramelize in the oven and turn into a sweet-tart edible treat. Cut oranges into ⅛-inch-thick "wagon wheel" slices, brush with olive oil, and roast for 25 minutes. Another favorite is roasted strawberries. Hull each berry and cut them in half, then place cut-side down on the parchment. Brush with olive oil and roast for 20 minutes.

Per Serving: Calories: 308; Total Fat: 19g; Saturated Fat: 5g; Cholesterol: 19mg; Sodium: 309mg; Total Carbohydrates: 29g; Fiber: 4g; Protein: 8g

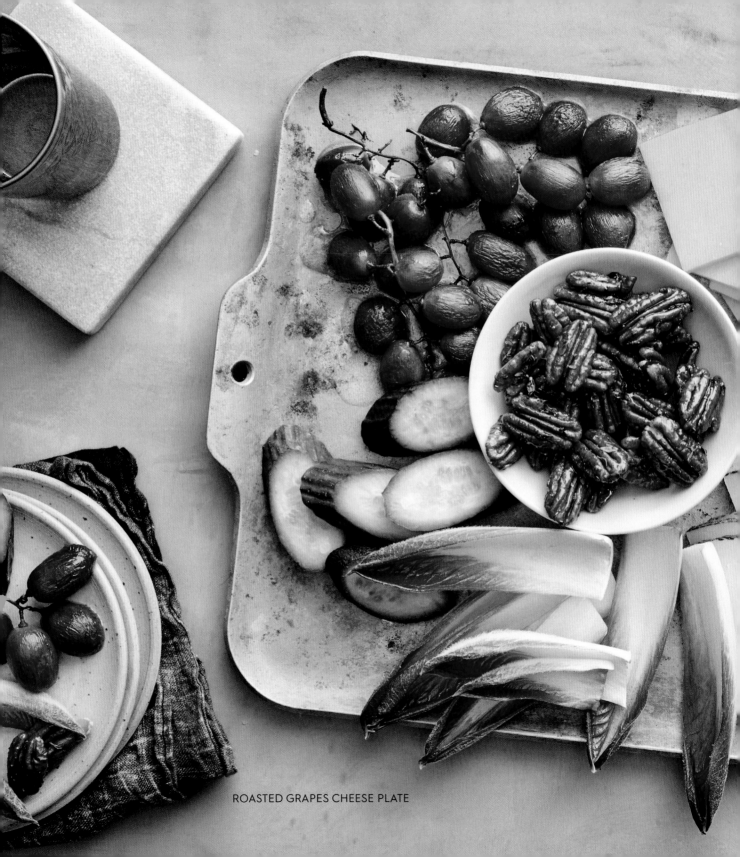

ROASTED GRAPES CHEESE PLATE

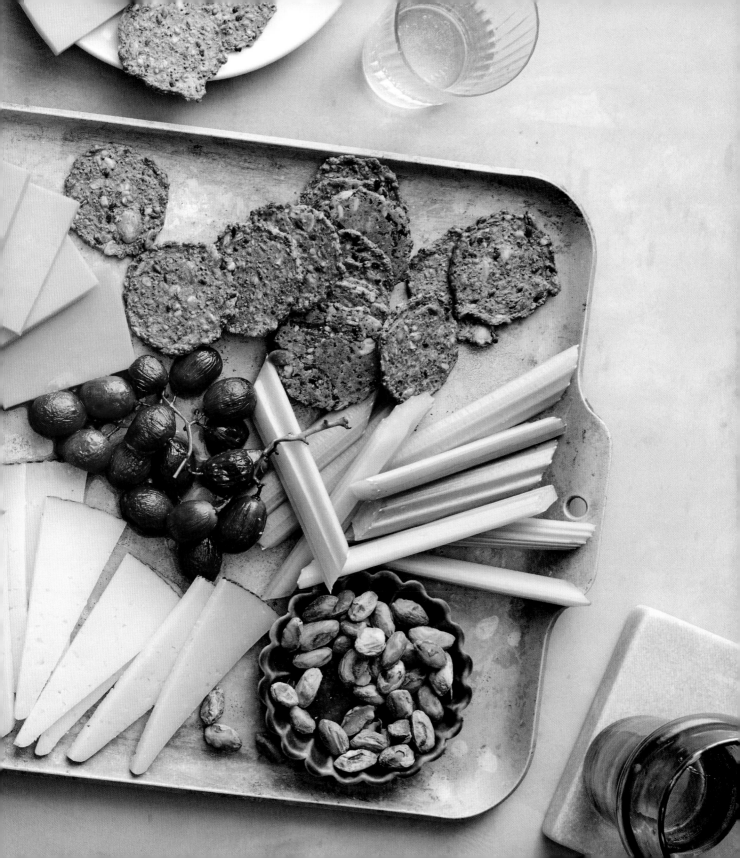

Htipiti (Whipped Feta and Red Pepper Spread) with Toasted Pita

| Nut-Free, Egg-Free, Vegetarian | Serves 8 | Prep time: 15 minutes |

6 ounces feta cheese, crumbled, rinsed if from a feta block (see Healthy Kitchen Hack below)

½ cup part-skim ricotta cheese (4 ounces)

1 whole roasted red pepper, store-bought or homemade (see page 44), drained and chopped

2 teaspoons honey

½ teaspoon black pepper

3 teaspoons extra-virgin olive oil, divided

1 medium lemon

⅓ cup chopped fresh chives or green onions

4 (6-inch) whole-wheat pita breads, torn into pieces

Htipiti is a traditional Greek feta cheese spread; its name means "beaten" in Greek. It's just as fun to pronounce (*htee-PEE-tee*) as it is to spread on fresh vegetables and warm pita bread. Serve it on a grazing board with a few other noshes like our Honey-Roasted Pecans with Thyme (page 41) and Spicy Sweet Quick Pickles (page 51).

Add the feta and ricotta to a food processor. (If you don't have a food processor, use an electric mixer or a whisk.) Pulse until well combined, stopping to scrape down the sides as necessary. Then puree for 30 seconds more until the mixture is whipped and slightly larger in volume. Add the roasted red pepper, honey, and black pepper to the whipped cheese. Turn on the processor and slowly pour in 2 teaspoons of the olive oil until well combined.

Place the whipped feta spread in a serving bowl and drizzle with the remaining 1 teaspoon olive oil. Grate half of the lemon zest with a Microplane or citrus zester over the top. (Save any remaining lemon for another use.) Sprinkle with the chives. Serve at room temperature with the pita bread pieces.

Healthy Kitchen Hack: We tested both types of feta in this recipe: crumbled feta and block feta. Generally, we prefer the creamier texture of block feta, but in this recipe, there wasn't a big taste difference. If you want to reduce the amount of sodium in your recipes, though, use block feta, as you can rinse away some of the salted brine with running water. Crumbled feta is coated in a powdered plant fiber (cellulose) to prevent clumping, so the rinsing trick doesn't work.

Per Serving: Calories: 177; Total Fat: 8g; Saturated Fat: 4g; Cholesterol: 24mg; Sodium: 402mg; Total Carbohydrates: 20g; Fiber: 2g; Protein: 8g

Parmesan Zucchini Chips

Nut-Free, Vegetarian	Serves 4	Prep time: 15 minutes	Cook time: 15 minutes

1 medium zucchini (about 5 ounces)

⅓ cup white whole-wheat flour

½ teaspoon smoked paprika

½ teaspoon garlic powder

¼ teaspoon kosher or sea salt

1 large egg, beaten

2 tablespoons water

½ cup panko breadcrumbs

3 tablespoons grated Parmesan cheese

1 tablespoon extra-virgin olive oil

Make a double batch of these chips because they might be the most delicious way to eat more veggies. Perfect for a party or a warm snack, our zuke chips are easier to master than traditional breaded veggies because the no-mess coating process will not result in sticky fingers by the end. (Serena developed it so she wouldn't have to clean up her kids after they help make these!)

Place a large rimmed baking sheet in the oven. Preheat the oven to 450°F.

On a cutting board, slice the zucchini into ¼-inch-thick coins. Set aside.

Into a gallon-size zip-top plastic bag, put the flour, smoked paprika, garlic powder, and salt. Shake the bag to combine the ingredients. Set aside.

In a medium bowl, whisk together the egg and water. Set aside.

Into another gallon-size zip-top plastic bag, put the breadcrumbs and Parmesan cheese. Shake the bag to combine the ingredients.

Place the zucchini coins into the bag with the flour mixture and shake it to coat all the pieces. Using a large slotted spoon, transfer the zucchini to the bowl with the egg mixture. Using a fork, gently toss the zucchini coins to coat them with the egg mixture. Using a large (clean) slotted spoon or a fork, lift the zucchini chips from the egg, allowing any extra coating to drip off, and then gently transfer them to the bag with the breadcrumb mixture. Shake the bag to coat all the coins.

Using oven mitts, carefully remove the baking sheet from the oven and add the olive oil. Tilt the pan to completely coat it with the oil.

Using tongs, remove the zucchini from the bag and place the coins on the baking sheet, making sure air can circulate between the pieces.

continued

Parmesan Zucchini Chips (continued)

Bake for 6 minutes, then remove the baking sheet from the oven. Turn the chips using a thin metal spatula. Bake for 6 minutes more, until the chips are golden brown.

Healthy Kitchen Hack: Use this breading technique to turn other vegetables into tasty snacks—try sliced eggplant, cauliflower pieces, broccoli florets, red pepper strips, or green beans. Use the breading amounts called for to coat about 4 cups veggies. If you double the recipe for larger amounts of vegetables, place no more than 4 cups of veggies in each bag or bowl at a time, otherwise the coating won't stick well.

Per Serving: Calories: 117; Total Fat: 6g; Saturated Fat: 2g; Cholesterol: 26mg; Sodium: 272mg; Total Carbohydrates: 12g; Fiber: 2g; Protein: 5g

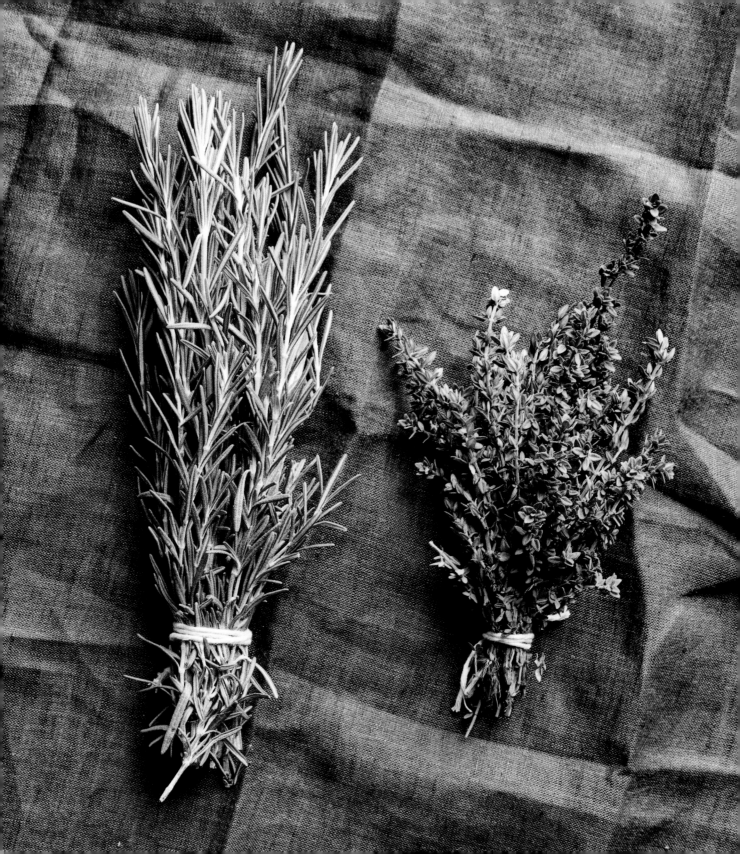

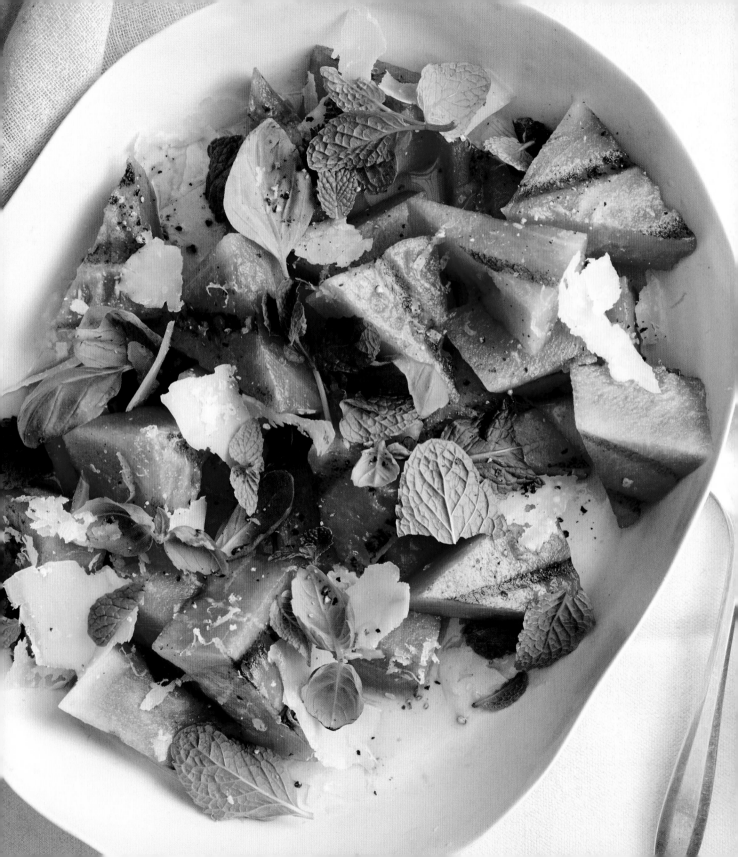

salads

Arugula with Apricot Balsamic Dressing

Dairy-Free, Gluten-Free, Egg-Free, Vegan | **Serves 4** | Prep time: 5 minutes | Cook time: 10 minutes

½ cup sliced almonds

1 (15-ounce) can apricot halves in light syrup, drained and rinsed

3 tablespoons extra-virgin olive oil

1 tablespoon regular or aged balsamic vinegar (see Healthy Kitchen Hack below)

¼ teaspoon kosher or sea salt

¼ teaspoon black pepper

6 cups arugula

Canned fruit is an absolute staple in our Mediterranean pantry for whipping up quick sauces, marinades, or dressings like this sweet and tangy vinaigrette made with drained and rinsed canned apricots. Don't limit its use to salad greens only! This recipe makes a double batch of dressing so you can also enjoy it as a flavor boost for baked or grilled chicken or a delicious topping for yogurt.

Heat a small skillet over medium heat and put the almonds in it. Cook, stirring occasionally, until the almonds are lightly toasted, 4 to 6 minutes, being careful not to burn them. Set aside.

Add the apricots, olive oil, vinegar, salt, and pepper to a blender. Blend until pureed.

Put the arugula and almonds in a large serving bowl. Right before serving, drizzle half of the dressing over the salad. Toss to serve. Store the remaining dressing in a sealed container in the refrigerator for up to 7 days.

Healthy Kitchen Hack: Aged balsamic vinegar is a tantalizingly acidic and sweet syrupy condiment used in many Italian dishes, yet it can be fairly expensive. You can make a similar version of it by adding ½ cup regular balsamic vinegar to a small saucepan. Cook it over medium-low heat for 15 minutes, stirring occasionally. Mix in 1 tablespoon honey and cook until the entire mixture reduces to about ¼ cup, 5 to 8 more minutes. Let it cool and then drizzle it over fresh fruit with herbs (try strawberries and mint!), toss it with green beans, or swirl it over vanilla ice cream.

Per Serving: Calories: 151; Total Fat: 11g; Saturated Fat: 1g; Cholesterol: 0mg; Sodium: 73mg; Total Carbohydrates: 11g; Fiber: 2g; Protein: 4g

Kale Caesar Salad with Chickpeas

Nut-Free, Egg-Free	Serves 8	Prep time: 15 minutes

1 garlic clove

1 small baguette, cut in half lengthwise, toasted, and cut into ½-inch cubes (about 2 cups)

1 (15-ounce) can chickpeas drained, 2 tablespoons of liquid reserved

1 medium lemon

2 tablespoons grated Parmesan cheese

1 tablespoon Dijon mustard

1 teaspoon Worcestershire sauce or less-sodium soy sauce

¼ teaspoon kosher or sea salt

¼ teaspoon black pepper

⅛ teaspoon crushed red pepper (optional)

3 tablespoons extra-virgin olive oil

10 cups chopped stemmed kale leaves

¼ cup shaved Parmesan or Pecorino Romano cheese

This modern twist on the classic Caesar salad leaves out the raw egg yolks and anchovies that are usually found in Caesar dressing. Worcestershire sauce or soy sauce adds back in the meaty or "umami" flavor. Switch up this recipe by mixing in different salad greens like romaine, arugula, or spinach, or tossing in different canned beans like cannellini, pinto, or kidney beans.

Cut the garlic clove in half. Rub one of the cut sides on both pieces of the toasted bread. Mince both garlic clove halves and set aside.

Rinse the chickpeas and pat dry with a paper towel or clean dish towel. Set aside.

To make the dressing, grate the lemon zest with a Microplane or citrus zester into a food processor or blender. Cut the lemon in half and squeeze 1 tablespoon of lemon juice into the food processor. (Save any remaining lemon for another use.) Add the garlic, reserved 2 tablespoons chickpea liquid, 2 tablespoons of the grated Parmesan cheese, the mustard, Worcestershire sauce, salt, black pepper, and (if desired) crushed red pepper. Process until pureed. While the food processor is running, slowly add the olive oil. Process until the dressing is smooth.

Put the kale and the chickpeas in a large serving bowl. Drizzle the dressing over the top and toss well. Let sit for 5 minutes for the dressing to slightly tenderize and soften the kale.

Top the salad with the toasted croutons and the shaved cheese, then toss again.

Healthy Kitchen Hack: For an upgrade to kale chips, roast this salad! Spread the dressed salad onto a large rimmed baking sheet. Cook in a preheated 400°F oven, stirring halfway, for about 15 minutes total, until the kale leaves crisp up.

Per Serving: Calories: 273; Total Fat: 9g; Saturated Fat: 2g; Cholesterol: 3mg; Sodium: 649mg; Total Carbohydrates: 38g; Fiber: 7g; Protein: 11g

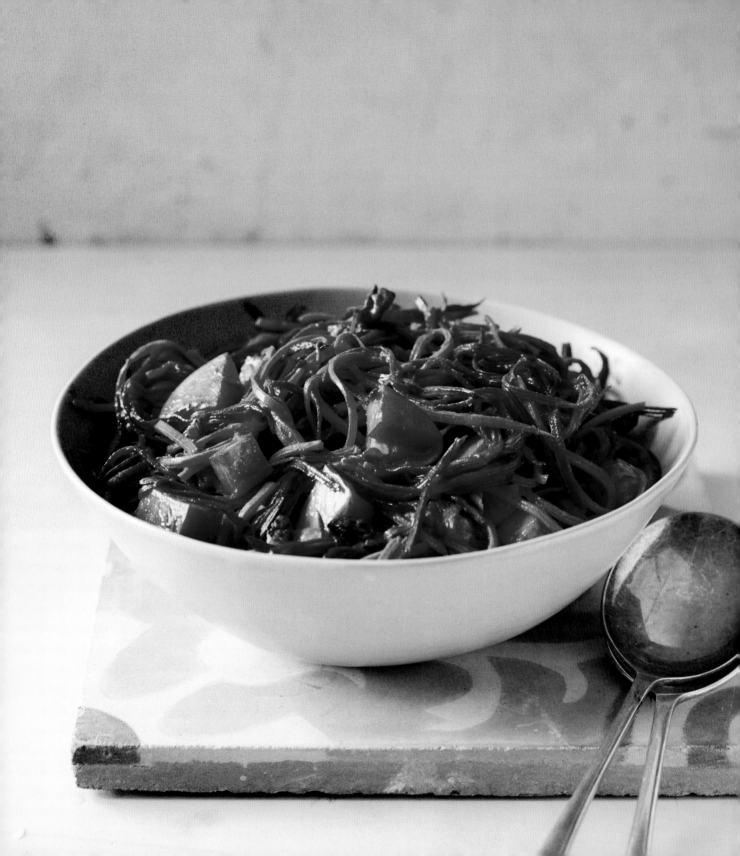

Shredded Beet-and-Apple Slaw

Gluten-Free, Egg-Free, Vegetarian	Serves 4	Prep time: 10 minutes

1 medium lemon, cut in half

½ cup plain 2% Greek yogurt

2 tablespoons honey

1 medium apple, chopped

1 medium beet, scrubbed

1 medium carrot, scrubbed

⅓ cup chopped pecans

¼ cup raisins

"I wasn't sure I would like raw beets, but I liked their crunch and sweetness, and so did my family. I subbed in walnuts instead of pecans and sour cream instead of Greek yogurt."

—PJ from La Grange, IL

In the Ball household, this is the go-to side for main dishes from Mediterranean Crispy Chicken and Potatoes (page 256) to pizza. Even Serena's kids can whip together this vibrant tangle of shredded root veggies with a touch of honeyed fruit. Raw beets and carrots are common in Mediterranean veggie dishes from Italy to Israel, as a tangy and delicious mix of sweet and sharp. And even in the dreary wintertime, bright orange carrots and ruby-red beets are in season when there isn't that much colorful fresh produce around.

Squeeze 1 tablespoon of lemon juice into a small bowl. (Save any remaining lemon for another use.) Add the yogurt and honey and whisk together. Add the chopped apple, mix together, and set aside.

Using the large holes on a box grater, shred the beet and the carrot. (For the most efficient shredding process, use long strokes as you run the vegetable from the top to the bottom of the grater. Other shredding options include using a mandoline or a julienne peeler.)

In a serving bowl, stir the shredded beet and carrot together. Add the yogurt mixture, pecans, and raisins. Stir to combine.

Healthy Kitchen Hack: To bump up the nutrition content, we don't peel the beet, carrot, or apple skins. Many of the phytonutrients—the components that help plants ward off disease and can help our bodies ward off disease, too—are located right beneath the skin. Peeling a fruit or vegetable strips these away.

Per Serving: Calories: 183; Total Fat: 7g; Saturated Fat: 1g; Cholesterol: 3mg; Sodium: 46mg; Total Carbohydrates: 30g; Fiber: 4g; Protein: 5g

Orange, Celery, and Olive Tabbouleh

Dairy-Free, Nut-Free, Egg-Free, Vegan	Serves 6	Prep time: 15 minutes	Cook time: 15 minutes

⅔ cup uncooked bulgur

¼ teaspoon kosher or sea salt

4 celery stalks, including their leaves

2 large oranges

⅓ cup canned or jarred pitted green olives, 2 tablespoons of liquid from the can or jar reserved

¼ cup thinly sliced red onion

1 medium lemon, cut in half

2 tablespoons extra-virgin olive oil

1 tablespoon Dijon mustard

¼ teaspoon black pepper

Tabbouleh is typically a combo of the whole grain bulgur, tomatoes, onions, mint, and parsley. But often we see versions with the fresh parsley as an afterthought instead of as the star ingredient in the true Mediterranean style of using an abundant amount of fresh herbs. Here we treat celery leaves the same way—not to be discarded but to be celebrated and used for their hearty flavor—in this sunny citrus-and-olive tabbouleh that will brighten your day.

Pour 1½ cups water into a medium saucepan and bring to a boil over medium heat. Stir in the bulgur and the salt; reduce the heat to medium-low. Cover and cook for 12 minutes. Remove from the heat, keep covered, and let stand for 10 minutes. Remove the lid and fluff with a fork. Scoop the bulgur onto a serving platter or into a large serving bowl.

While the bulgur cooks, slice the celery stalks into ½-inch slices and chop the leaves. Peel the oranges and pull each apart so you have two halves for each. Slice each half into ¼-inch-thick slices. Toss the celery, oranges, green olives, and onions over the bulgur.

Squeeze 2 tablespoons of lemon juice into a small bowl. (Save any remaining lemon for another use.) Add the olive oil, liquid from the green olives, mustard, and black pepper and whisk together. Pour the dressing over the bulgur salad and toss gently.

Healthy Kitchen Hack: We love celery leaves! Compared to celery hearts, buying the entire head of celery (with the stalks and leaves attached) is more budget-friendly and also way more flavorful. Celery leaves have a bold taste that means a richer antioxidant content—a win-win! In addition to grain dishes, add celery leaves to soups, green salads, potato salads, and tuna sandwiches.

Per Serving: Calories: 146; Total Fat: 7g; Saturated Fat: 2g; Cholesterol: 0mg; Sodium: 246mg; Total Carbohydrates: 20g; Fiber: 4g; Protein: 3g

Peach-Avocado Caprese Plate

Nut-Free, Gluten-Free, Egg-Free, Vegetarian	Serves 6	Prep time: 15 minutes

2 large tomatoes, cut into ¼-inch slices

2 medium peaches, pitted and cut into ¼-inch slices

2 large fresh mozzarella balls (about 8 ounces total), cut into ¼-inch slices

1 avocado, pitted, peeled, and cut in ¼-inch slices

¼ cup fresh basil leaves, torn

2 tablespoons extra-virgin olive oil

1 tablespoon balsamic vinegar

¼ teaspoon kosher or sea salt

¼ teaspoon black pepper

When warmer weather hits, Deanna's go-to side dish is ripe tomatoes, fresh mozzarella, and sweet basil mixed with olive oil and salt—the traditional caprese salad. Every summer, she likes to experiment with different variations on this salad, and this one with avocados and peaches is her favorite result to date. Since avocados are usually available year-round, she even whips this up in the winter months using canned peaches and grape tomatoes to conjure up some Mediterranean sunshine in her Philadelphia kitchen.

On a large serving platter, alternate tomato slices, peach slices, mozzarella slices, avocado slices, and torn basil leaves in rows with each piece slightly overlapping. Immediately before serving, drizzle the salad with the olive oil and vinegar. Sprinkle with the salt and black pepper.

Healthy Kitchen Hack: Make a panini sandwich out of the leftovers! Brush two slices of whole-grain or Italian bread with olive oil. Place a small portion of the salad between the bread and place the sandwich in a large nonstick skillet over medium heat. Add a weighted object such as another skillet or a tea kettle (as Deanna uses) on top of the sandwich to press the sandwich as it cooks. Cook for 4 to 5 minutes per side until golden brown and the cheese is melted.

Per Serving: Calories: 220; Total Fat: 16g; Saturated Fat: 5g; Cholesterol: 13mg; Sodium: 303mg; Total Carbohydrates: 11g; Fiber: 4g; Protein: 10g

Grilled Watermelon Salad

Nut-Free, Gluten-Free, Egg-Free, Vegetarian	Serves 6	Prep time: 15 minutes	Cook time: 20 minutes

1 small seedless watermelon (5 to 6 pounds)

1½ tablespoons extra-virgin olive oil

1 medium lemon

¼ cup fresh basil leaves, torn

¼ cup fresh mint leaves, torn

⅓ cup shaved Parmesan cheese (about 1½ ounces)

⅛ teaspoon black pepper

Throwing watermelon slices on the grill may seem odd, but after the first time Serena tried this, she was hooked. Much like roasting other fruits (see our Roasted Grapes Cheese Plate on page 53), grilling watermelon enhances the fruit's natural sugars. Tossed with salty Parmesan and fresh sweet herbs, this memorable salad is perfect for hot summer days and outdoor celebrations.

Preheat a grill to medium-high or heat a grill pan over medium-high heat.

Cut the watermelon in half from the stem to the bottom. Cut each half in half again. Cut each quarter into ¾-inch-thick slices. Brush both sides of each slice with olive oil.

Grill the watermelon in batches until grill marks appear, 2 to 3 minutes per side.

Remove the watermelon slices and cool for 10 minutes. Cut off the rinds (but don't discard them—see the Healthy Kitchen Hack below) and chop the watermelon into 1½- to 2-inch chunks. Put the chunks into a large serving bowl.

Grate the lemon zest with a Microplane or citrus zester into the bowl. Cut the lemon in half and squeeze in the juice from one half. (Save the remaining lemon half for another use.) Add the basil, mint, shaved cheese, and black pepper. Toss gently until all the ingredients are well mixed. If there is excess watermelon juice in the bowl before serving, drain the salad in a colander over the sink and then return the salad to the bowl.

Healthy Kitchen Hack: Did you know you can eat the watermelon rind? We're talking about the white part between the red flesh and the tough green skin, which typically gets tossed. After cutting up your watermelon, slice the white rind away from the green skin. Cube the rind and toss it with your favorite salad greens or cut into matchstick pieces and toss it into a slaw (like our Shredded Beet-and-Apple Slaw on page 65). You can even sauté it like zucchini—it will have a similar texture and flavor to that of cooked summer squash.

Per Serving: Calories: 115; Total Fat: 6g; Saturated Fat: 2g; Total Carbohydrates: 25g; Fiber: 2g; Cholesterol: 6mg; Sodium: 131mg; Protein: 4g

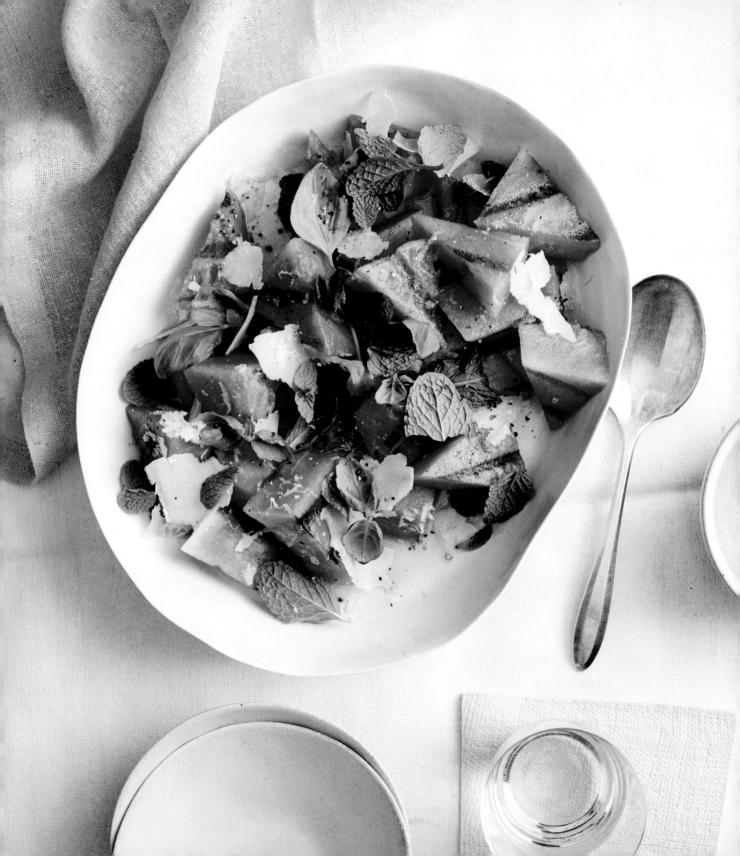

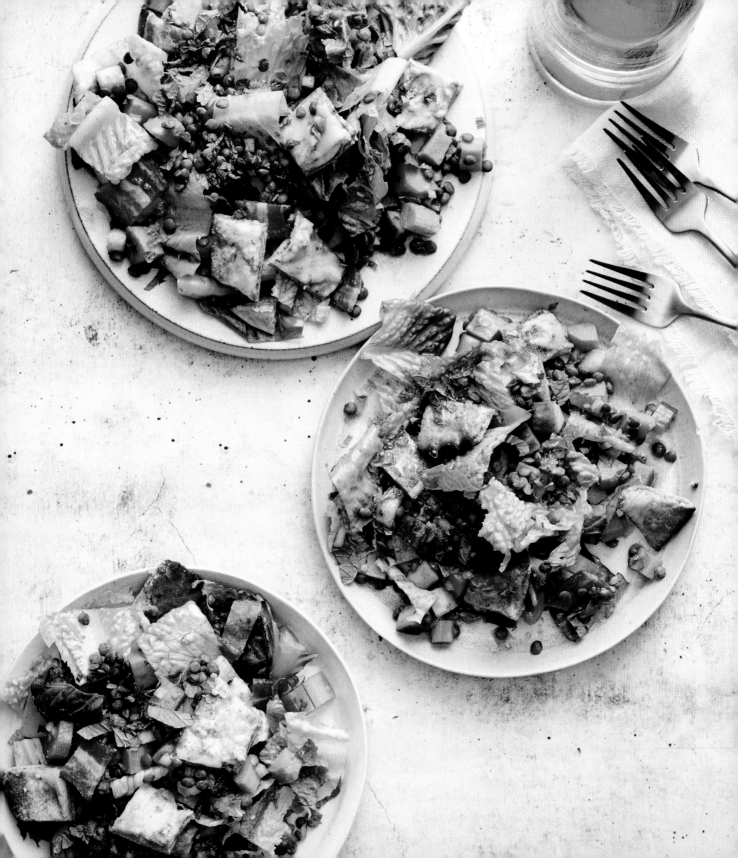

Lentil-Bacon Fattoush Salad with Gorgonzola Pita

Nut-Free, Egg-Free		Serves 8	Prep time: 10 minutes	Cook time: 25 minutes

¾ cup uncooked brown or green lentils

1¼ cups low-sodium or no-salt-added vegetable broth

3 pieces center-cut bacon

2 (6-inch) whole-wheat pita breads

½ cup crumbled Gorgonzola cheese (2 ounces)

1 medium lemon

⅓ cup extra-virgin olive oil

1 teaspoon honey

½ teaspoon za'atar or dried thyme

1 romaine head, chopped (about 4½ cups)

2 large carrots, chopped (about 1 cup)

1 large seedless cucumber, chopped (about 1 cup)

½ red onion, minced (about ½ cup)

⅓ cup fresh mint, chopped

Fattoush is a classic Lebanese salad featuring toasted flatbread, chopped vegetables, and fresh herbs. This hearty version is rich in protein, fiber, iron, folate and flavor. Serve it as a main meal or as a side dish to our Microwave Salmon with Green Onions (page 168) or White Wine-Roasted Chicken with Apples (page 258).

Preheat the oven to 425°F. Line a large rimmed baking sheet with aluminum foil.

Into a medium saucepan, put the lentils and broth and bring to a boil over high heat. Cover the pan and reduce the heat to low. Cook until the broth is absorbed and the lentils are tender, 22 to 25 minutes. (Note: Check the saucepan about 5 minutes before done to make sure enough liquid remains to prevent the lentils from burning before they are fully cooked.) Remove from heat.

While the lentils are cooking, arrange the bacon on the foil-lined pan. Bake for 12 to 14 minutes until the bacon is golden brown and crisp to your liking. Remove from the oven and, using tongs, place the bacon on paper towels to absorb the grease. Once the bacon is cool to the touch, tear or cut it into bite-size pieces. Set aside.

Turn the oven to the broiler setting.

Remove the foil from the baking sheet. Place the pitas on the pan in a single layer and sprinkle with the Gorgonzola. Broil, watching closely to keep the pita from burning, for 1½ to 2 minutes or until the cheese is melted. Place on a cutting board and, using a pizza cutter or knife, slice into 1-inch square bites. Set aside.

Grate the lemon zest with a Microplane or a zester into a small bowl. Cut the lemon in half and squeeze 3 tablespoons of lemon juice into the bowl. (Save any remaining lemon for another use.) Add the olive oil, honey, and za'atar. Whisk together to create a dressing.

continued

Lentil-Bacon Fattoush Salad with Gorgonzola Pita (continued)

In a large serving bowl, put the lettuce, carrots, cucumber, onion, cooked lentils, bacon, and pita bites. Drizzle with the dressing and toss well. Sprinkle with the mint and serve.

Healthy Kitchen Hack: Bacon may seem out of place when talking about healthy eats, but cured meats play a role in Mediterranean cuisine—the key is that a little goes a long way. Look for center-cut bacon, which contains more pork meat and less fat. If you have more time in the kitchen, start the bacon in a cold oven. Turn the oven temperature to 400°F and cook until the bacon is crisp to your liking, about 20 minutes. The slow rise in heat helps render more fat from the bacon.

Per Serving: Calories: 262; Total Fat: 13g; Saturated Fat: 3g; Cholesterol: 8mg; Sodium: 271mg; Total Carbohydrates: 28g; Fiber: 6g; Protein: 10g

"I'd never used za'atar before and the next time I make this, I'll add even more! I also loved the pita crisps and the fresh mint. The leftovers made for a delicious lunch the next day."

—Sharon from Madison Heights, MI

Herb Salad with Citrus-Date Dressing

Dairy-Free, Nut-Free, Gluten-Free, Egg-Free, Vegan	Serves 4	Prep time: 15 minutes

4 whole Deglet Noor dates or 2 Medjool dates, pitted

4 cups mixed salad greens

2 cups chopped fresh parsley or cilantro

2 medium lemons, cut in half

1 large orange, cut in half

1 tablespoon Dijon mustard

¼ teaspoon kosher or sea salt

¼ teaspoon black pepper

3 tablespoons extra-virgin olive oil

Optional add-ins: roasted vegetables, aged cheese, aged salami, Cinnamon-Spiced Sweet Potato Wedges (page 83), or Honey-Roasted Pecans with Thyme (page 41)

Dates are the "secret" ingredient in this multidimensionally flavored dressing. While Medjool dates (the sticky-sweet dates found in plastic containers in the produce department) are a popular natural sweetener in smoothies, energy bars, and baked goods, we like to use Deglet Noor dates. They are just as versatile, a bit less sticky, and definitely less expensive. We use them here to sweeten the only homemade dressing so far that has gotten Serena's kids to eat green salad.

Fill a small bowl with ¼ cup hot water and add the dates. Let set for 5 minutes to soften.

Into a large serving bowl, put the greens and parsley. Toss to combine.

Squeeze 3 tablespoons of lemon juice and 3 tablespoons of orange juice into a blender. (Save any remaining lemon or orange juice for another use.) Add the soaked dates and their liquid, mustard, salt, and black pepper. Puree to combine. With the motor running, drizzle in the olive oil.

Pour half of the dressing over the greens and toss to coat, then serve. Save the remaining dressing for another use, or if you add any or all of the optional add-ins, use more dressing to taste.

Healthy Kitchen Hack: Move this salad out of the "sides" department and into the "mains." By adding your favorite cooked protein like leftover chicken, cooked shrimp, canned tuna, or canned chickpeas, you'll have a main dish ready in minutes.

Per Serving: Calories: 138; Total Fat: 11g; Saturated Fat: 2g; Cholesterol: 0mg; Sodium: 300mg; Total Carbohydrates: 10g; Fiber: 2g; Protein: 2g

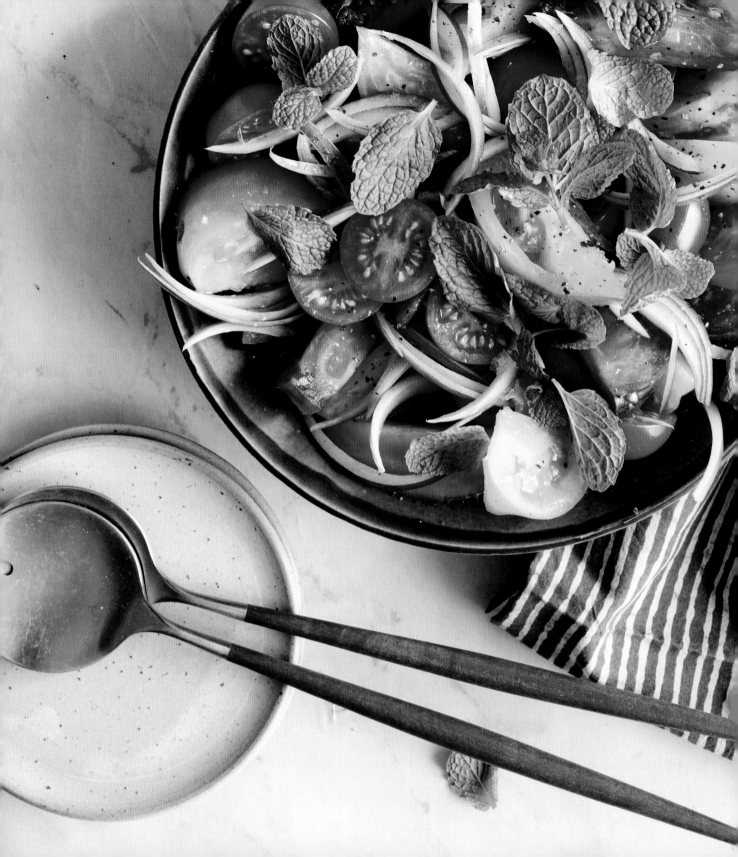

sides

Charred Green Beans with Za'atar

Dairy-Free, Nut-Free, Gluten-Free, Egg-Free, Vegan	Serves 4	Prep time: 5 minutes	Cook time: 10 minutes

1 pound green beans, trimmed

½ medium red onion, thinly sliced (about ½ cup)

2 tablespoons extra-virgin olive oil, divided

1 medium lemon, cut in half

½ teaspoon za'atar

Deanna was never a huge fan of green beans until she had them charred under a broiler. Now it's about the only way she'll cook them. Since her trip to Israel, she uses za'atar often and found it to be the perfect complement to green beans. If she has extra grape tomatoes on hand, she mixes them in with the rest of the ingredients before it all goes into the oven, which gives a pop of color and a hint of sweetness.

Preheat the broiler to high.

Into a large serving bowl, put the green beans, onion, and 1 tablespoon of the olive oil. Using your hands, mix until the vegetables are well coated. Spread the bean mixture out onto a large rimmed baking sheet. Broil, stirring twice, for 6 to 8 minutes, until the beans are slightly blackened and tender. Remove from the oven.

While the beans cook, squeeze 1 tablespoon of lemon juice into a small bowl. (Save any remaining lemon for another use.) Add the remaining 1 tablespoon olive oil and the za'atar; whisk until well blended.

Put the charred beans back into the serving bowl. Drizzle with the za'atar dressing and serve warm.

Healthy Kitchen Hack: Use this charring technique—a blast of high heat—to quickly cook just about any veggie. Delicate vegetables like zucchini and tomatoes will char faster than root and cruciferous vegetables like carrots, cabbage, and broccoli. Make sure your veggies are cut in similar sizes to avoid a combination of burnt and undercooked pieces when serving.

Per Serving: Calories: 105; Total Fat: 7g; Saturated Fat: 1g; Cholesterol: 0mg; Sodium: 16mg; Total Carbohydrates: 10g; Fiber: 4g; Protein: 2g

Roasted Butternut Squash with Cilantro-Olive Salsa

Dairy-Free, Nut-Free, Gluten-Free, Egg-Free, Vegan	Serves 6	Prep time: 10 minutes	Cook time: 20 minutes

1 butternut squash (about 3 pounds)

1 tablespoon plus 2 teaspoons extra-virgin olive oil, divided

1 cup chopped fresh cilantro

⅓ cup chopped green olives from a jar, ¼ cup liquid reserved

¼ cup minced red onion

1 garlic clove, minced

1 tablespoon red wine vinegar

¼ teaspoon crushed red pepper

We want to take you beyond the typical brown sugar–topped cooked squash. Fresh from the Israeli table, this is a savory way to enjoy squash, including a bright cilantro-olive sauce. We love cilantro but understand not everyone does, so feel free to swap in parsley, chives, mint, or any combo of fresh herbs you have on hand. This salsa is so good we had to use it in our Marinara Chicken-Lentil Bake (page 261), too.

Preheat the oven to 400°F. Line a large rimmed baking sheet with aluminum foil or parchment paper.

Rinse the butternut squash to remove any dirt. Using a sharp paring knife, poke a few holes in the squash to release steam. Microwave the squash on high for 5 minutes.

Using oven mitts, remove the squash from the microwave, place it on a cutting board, and let it cool slightly. Slice a thin strip off the side to make a flat surface. Lay the squash on that flat surface and peel it using a vegetable peeler. Cut the squash in half lengthwise. Scrape out the seeds using a large spoon. (Reserve the seeds to roast!) Slice the squash into half-moon slices about ¾ inch thick. Brush both sides of the squash with 2 teaspoons of the olive oil and place on the prepared baking sheet.

Roast for about 15 minutes or until the squash slices have softened. (If you prefer golden brown squash, roast for 5 to 10 more minutes.)

As the squash cooks, make the salsa. In a medium bowl, add the remaining 1 tablespoon olive oil, the cilantro, olives, olive liquid, onion, garlic, vinegar, and crushed red pepper.

To serve, place the squash on a serving platter and spoon the salsa over the squash.

continued

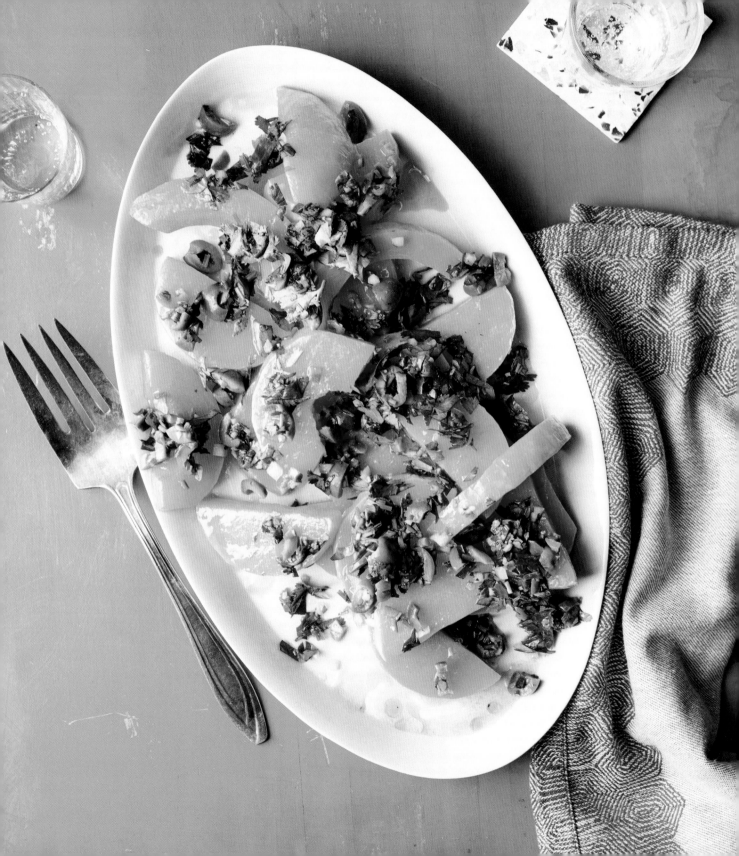

Roasted Butternut Squash with Cilantro-Olive Salsa (continued)

Healthy Kitchen Hack: You can use the microwave-softening method described in the recipe directions for easy slicing of any thick-skinned winter squash—like acorn, kabocha, or spaghetti squash. Microwaving the whole squash first also cuts in half the typical time it takes to roast squash in the oven. After cutting your squash, you can even skip oven roasting altogether and finish cooking it in the microwave to save even more time.

Per Serving: Calories: 136; Total Fat: 5g; Saturated Fat: 0g; Cholesterol: 0mg; Sodium: 357mg; Total Carbohydrates: 25g; Fiber: 4g; Protein: 2g

"I ate the squash the night I made it and then again the next morning for breakfast—so good, good, good! There were lots of veggie breakfast dishes like this when I visited Israel and Egypt, served both hot and cold."

—Candice from Alhambra, IL

Cheesy Cauliflower and Green Onion Gratinati

| Nut-Free, Egg-Free, Vegetarian | Serves 6 | Prep time: 5 minutes | Cook time: 25 minutes |

1 medium lemon

3 green onions, thinly sliced

¾ cup part-skim ricotta cheese

½ teaspoon garlic powder

¼ teaspoon kosher or sea salt

¼ teaspoon black pepper

2 (12-ounce) packages frozen cauliflower

¼ cup panko breadcrumbs

¼ cup grated Parmesan or Pecorino Romano cheese

A gratin is topped with cheese and breadcrumbs, then heated under the broiler until the top is browned and crispy. *Au gratin* is the French version but we think the Italian *gratinati* is even more fun to say. This crunchy topping can make any Mediterranean vegetable more enticing—and it even works with frozen veggies. Here we use frozen cauliflower, but frozen broccoli, frozen mixed veggies, or frozen diced hash brown potatoes would also be delish.

Place an oven rack about 4 inches below the broiler and place another rack in the middle of the oven. Preheat the oven to 400°F.

Using a Microplane or citrus zester, grate the zest of the lemon into a medium bowl. Stir in the green onions, ricotta, garlic powder, salt, and black pepper. Set aside.

Coat an 8- or 9-inch square glass baking dish with cooking spray. Place the frozen cauliflower in the prepared baking dish. Cut the lemon in half and squeeze about 1 tablespoon of lemon juice over the cauliflower. (Save any remaining lemon for another use.) Drizzle the cauliflower with ⅓ cup water. Cover with a paper towel and microwave on high, stirring halfway through, until the cauliflower is no longer icy, about 8 minutes.

While the cauliflower microwaves, add the panko breadcrumbs and Parmesan cheese to a medium bowl and stir.

Scoop the ricotta mixture onto the thawed cauliflower and mix to coat. Bake on the middle rack for 15 minutes until the cauliflower has softened. Remove the cauliflower from the oven and turn on the broiler.

Sprinkle the Parmesan mixture over the top of the cauliflower and broil for 2 minutes. Carefully turn the dish and then broil for another 1 to 2 minutes until the top is golden brown.

Healthy Kitchen Hack: The terms "green onions," "scallions," and "chives" can be confusing. Green onions and scallions are used interchangeably, but chives are a fresh herb. To use up any leftover green onions (or scallions!), chop and toss them chopped into pasta or puree them with olive oil and vinegar for a vinaigrette. Grill or sauté whole scallions until they turn silky-sweet, then add them to grain bowls or use as a pizza topping.

Per Serving: Calories: 95; Total Fat: 4g; Saturated Fat: 2g; Cholesterol: 12mg; Sodium: 200mg; Total Carbohydrates: 10g; Fiber: 3g; Protein: 7g

"Ricotta is one of my favorite cheeses, and the lemon really keeps the whole dish tasting fresh. I also like that this dish features affordable ingredients and is fast and easy to make."

—Ashley from Pittsburgh, PA

Easy Broccoli with Toasted Spices

Dairy-Free, Nut-Free, Gluten-Free, Egg-Free, Vegetarian	Serves 4	Prep time: 5 minutes	Cook time: 10 minutes

1 pound fresh broccoli (about 2 heads with stems)

1½ tablespoons extra-virgin olive oil

4 garlic cloves, minced

½ teaspoon fennel seeds (or see spice options in Healthy Kitchen Hack below)

⅛ to ¼ teaspoon crushed red pepper (depending on heat level desired)

1 teaspoon honey

¼ teaspoon kosher or sea salt

Broccoli sautéed in garlic-scented olive oil is one of our favorite ways to make this ho-hum vegetable become a craveable side dish. Adding the salt at the end means your tongue will taste it first and there will seem to be more salt than the meager quarter teaspoon used. A drizzle of honey is the magical ingredient to tie together the savory garlic, toasted spices, salt, and slightly bitter veggie into one irresistible bite.

Cut the broccoli into florets about 1 inch in size. Do not discard the leaves or stem. Slice off any tough peel on the stem, then slice it into ½-inch-thick rounds. Set aside.

Heat a large skillet over medium-high heat and pour in the olive oil. Add the garlic, fennel, and crushed red pepper and cook, stirring constantly to prevent burning, for 1 minute.

Add the broccoli and broccoli leaves and stems to the skillet and cook, stirring often to keep the garlic from burning, until the broccoli has slightly softened with a few darkly toasted edges, about 5 minutes. Remove from the heat. Drizzle with the honey and sprinkle with the salt. Toss to combine and serve.

Healthy Kitchen Hack: We use the method of toasting spices known as "blooming" in this dish. Heating the spices in oil infuses their fat-soluble flavors much better than infusing into water. Also, these aromatic oils distribute flavor throughout a dish better than almost any other way of adding spices. Besides the sweet-and-savory anise-flavored fennel seeds we use here, many other whole or ground spices would be delicious, like cumin and coriander seeds, mustard seeds and crushed red pepper, or ground cinnamon and ground cumin.

Per Serving: Calories: 95; Total Fat: 6g; Saturated Fat: 1g; Cholesterol: 0mg; Sodium: 158mg; Total Carbohydrates: 10g; Fiber: 3g; Protein: 3g

Cinnamon-Spiced Sweet Potato Wedges

Gluten-Free, Egg-Free, Vegetarian	Serves 6	Prep time: 10 minutes	Cook time: 20 minutes

1 tablespoon extra-virgin olive oil

1 teaspoon ground cinnamon

1 teaspoon ground cumin, divided

½ teaspoon ground ginger

¼ teaspoon kosher or sea salt

¼ teaspoon black pepper

1 pound sweet potatoes (about 3 small)

1 medium orange

1 tablespoon peanut butter

½ cup plain 2% Greek yogurt (4 ounces)

1 tablespoon honey

Two people asked Serena for this recipe when she took these to a party—and the sweet potatoes weren't even hot and crispy out of the oven. These sweet potato "fries" are snackable at any temperature. The nut butter dip is optional, but the combo of peanut butter, cumin, and cinnamon adds a tasty North African touch. We also think you'll find our slicing technique much easier than most homemade fries' recipes.

Preheat the oven to 425°F. Place a large rimmed baking sheet in the oven to heat.

Into a large bowl, put the olive oil, cinnamon, ½ teaspoon of the cumin, the ginger, salt, and black pepper. Set aside.

Slice each sweet potato in half. Place each half cut-side down and make ¼-inch-thick slices. (The slices will be different sizes, but the same thickness.) Add to the large bowl and toss to coat with the oil-spice mixture.

Carefully remove the hot baking sheet from the oven and place the potatoes evenly over the pan. Bake, flipping halfway through, for a total of about 20 minutes or until golden.

While the potatoes are baking, using a Microplane or citrus zester, grate the zest from about half the orange into a medium serving bowl. Cut the orange in half and squeeze 2 tablespoons of orange juice into the bowl. (Save any remaining orange for another use.) Add the peanut butter, yogurt, honey, and remaining ½ teaspoon cumin and whisk to combine.

Serve the sweet potato wedges right out of the oven with the dipping sauce.

Healthy Kitchen Hack: Throughout this book we use peanut butter and tahini in several sauces. If you have trouble incorporating these thick and sticky ingredients into a mixture, stir them first with a tablespoon of very hot or boiling water. This will soften some of the oils to allow the paste to mix in easier.

Per Serving: Calories: 130; Total Fat: 4g; Saturated Fat: 1g; Cholesterol: 2mg; Sodium: 140mg; Total Carbohydrates: 21g; Fiber: 3g; Protein: 4g

Israeli Roasted Eggplant

Nut-Free, Gluten-Free, Egg-Free, Vegetarian	Serves 4	Prep time: 5 minutes	Cook time: 30 minutes

2 medium eggplants, cut in half lengthwise

¼ cup olive oil, divided

1 teaspoon za'atar, divided

¼ teaspoon kosher or sea salt

½ cup plain 2% Greek yogurt (about 4 ounces)

1 (12-ounce) jar roasted red peppers or 2 Roasted Red Peppers (page 44), drained and chopped

2 teaspoons honey

¼ cup chopped fresh parsley

"I really liked the za'atar spice and the honey drizzle on top. I'd love to try to make this on the grill!"

—Aileen from Warrington, PA

Before visiting Israel, Deanna's primary exposure to eggplant was via Italian cuisine. But one of her favorite food experiences during her trip through Israel was all the glorious ways eggplant was prepared and served at every meal, even breakfast! This attractive dish is a mash-up of a few of the different preparations she enjoyed there. She shares even more options for how to serve it in the Healthy Kitchen Hacks below.

Preheat the oven to 425°F. Line a large rimmed baking sheet with aluminum foil. Place each eggplant half on the baking sheet, cut-side up.

In a small bowl, whisk together 3 tablespoons of the olive oil, ½ teaspoon of the za'atar, the salt, then brush over each eggplant half. Roast the eggplant for 28 to 30 minutes, until the eggplant flesh is very soft. Remove from the oven and set the pan on a wire rack.

While the eggplant cooks, in a small bowl, whisk together the yogurt, remaining 1 tablespoon olive oil, and remaining ½ teaspoon za'atar. Whisk in 2 tablespoons water to create a pourable sauce.

Spoon the yogurt sauce over each eggplant half and top each with the chopped roasted peppers. Drizzle with the honey. Top with the parsley.

Healthy Kitchen Hack: There are endless, delish ways to top roasted eggplant (all of which Deanna got to sample in Israel) including canned chickpeas, tahini, hummus, chopped tomatoes, pesto, sesame seeds, and pomegranate seeds. Also, be sure to try our Smoky Baba Ghanoush Dip on page 49 (another topping idea!), which includes a quick-cook method for eggplant using your broiler.

Per Serving: Calories: 238; Total Fat: 15g; Saturated Fat: 3g; Cholesterol: 3mg; Sodium: 461mg; Total Carbohydrates: 27g; Fiber: 8g; Protein: 6g

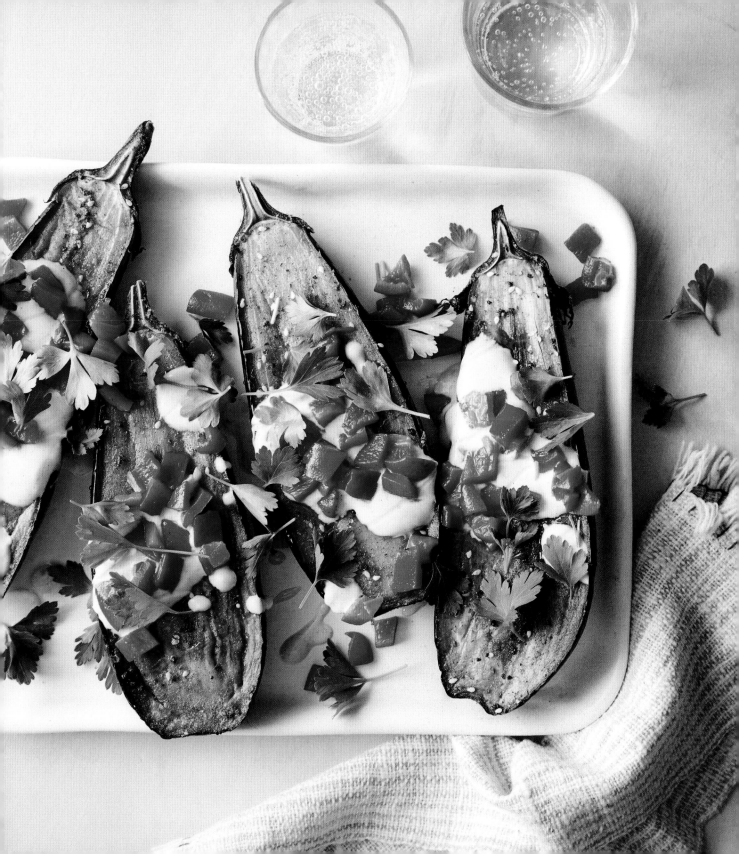

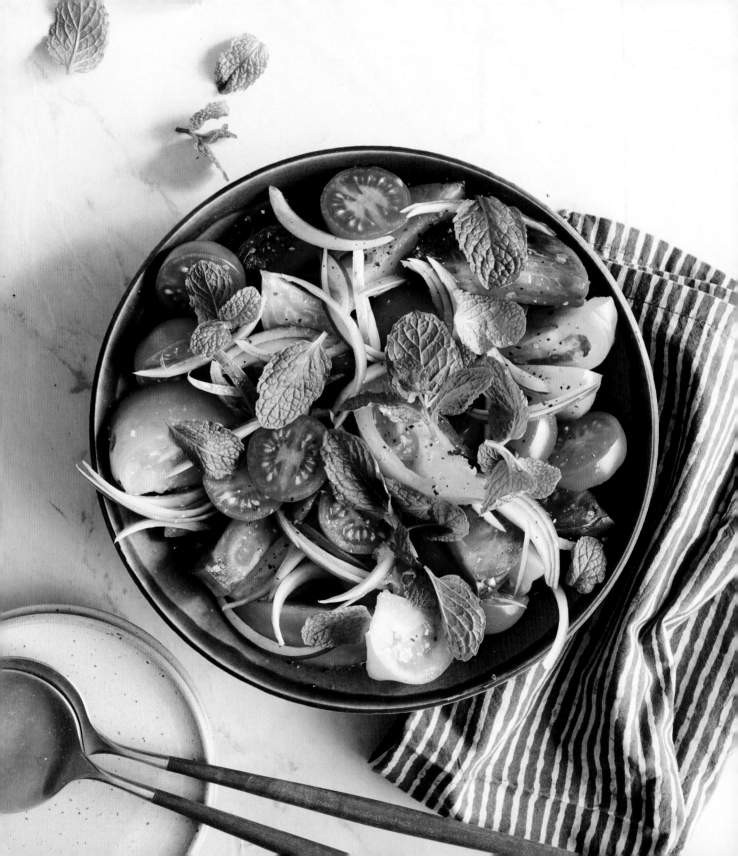

Tomato-Onion Plate with Mint

Dairy-Free, Nut-Free, Gluten-Free, Egg-Free, Vegetarian	Serves 6	Prep time: 20 minutes

3 large tomatoes

½ small red or sweet onion, thinly sliced

3 tablespoons extra-virgin olive oil

1½ tablespoons red wine vinegar or white wine vinegar

1 teaspoon honey

¼ teaspoon kosher or sea salt

¼ teaspoon black pepper

3 tablespoons fresh mint leaves

In the true spirit of the Mediterranean way of eating, this dish is simple, seasonal, and super good. Both Deanna's Nana and Serena's Grandma made a similar side dish every summer without fail when their garden tomatoes were at their peak. Deanna likes to do a mix of red onions with sweet white onions to add different colors and flavors. The dark green fresh mint topping adds a contrasting color and a hint of sweet, making this an essential hot-weather cooling side dish.

Cut the tomatoes into wedges or slices. Arrange on a serving platter. Spread the onion over top. Set aside.

Into a small bowl, measure the olive oil, vinegar, honey, salt, and black pepper. Whisk together and then drizzle over the tomatoes and onion. Let sit for at least 10 minutes before serving. Right before serving, tear the mint leaves and sprinkle them over the salad.

If making the salad ahead of time, mix all the ingredients together except for the mint and store in the refrigerator. Let the salad come to room temperature before serving (and don't forget to add the mint!).

Healthy Kitchen Hack: Raw red onions add incredible color to dishes but also add a lot of bite (and let's face it, they don't give you the best breath either). To cut back on that sharp flavor, soak your cut onions in an ice-water bath for about 15 minutes. The water will help wash away a lot of the sulfur compounds that give raw onions their strong taste.

Per Serving: Calories: 127; Total Fat: 11g; Saturated Fat: 2g; Cholesterol: 0mg; Sodium: 129mg; Total Carbohydrates: 8g; Fiber: 2g; Protein: 2g

Red Potatoes with Mint Pesto

| Gluten-Free, Egg-Free, Vegetarian | Serves 8 | Prep time: 10 minutes | Cook time: 20 minutes |

2 cups frozen green peas, divided

2½ pounds red potatoes

2 cups chopped fresh parsley

1 cup chopped fresh mint leaves

¼ cup shredded Parmesan or Pecorino Romano cheese (1 ounce)

⅓ cup chopped walnuts

1 garlic clove

¼ teaspoon kosher or sea salt

3 tablespoons extra-virgin olive oil

When Serena was a child, one of the most highly anticipated dishes from her father's giant vegetable garden was "creamed peas and new potatoes." This spring dish is loosely based on that classic combo of peas and potatoes. But we also like to make any pesto with peas to bump up the nutrition and the bright green color. If you've ever had a basil pesto turn a drab olive-green on you, add thawed frozen peas. They will keep the sauce that gorgeous, vivid green color.

Place the peas on the counter to thaw.

Cut the potatoes into 1-inch cubes. Place them in a medium saucepan and add cold water to cover them by 1 inch. Bring the water to a boil over high heat. Once the water boils, reduce the heat to medium and cook until the potatoes just start to feel soft when tested with a fork, about 12 minutes. Add 1 cup of the peas to the pan and then immediately drain the potatoes and peas.

While the potatoes are cooking, in a food processor, put the parsley, mint, cheese, walnuts, garlic, and salt and pulse until roughly chopped (about ten times). Scrape down the sides of the processor, add the remaining 1 cup peas and pulse until roughly chopped. Scrape down the sides. Turn the processor on and drizzle in the olive oil. Once the oil has been added, immediately turn off the processor so the pesto remains slightly chunky.

Place the potatoes and peas in a serving bowl, then add the pesto and toss gently to coat. Serve at room temperature.

Healthy Kitchen Hack: One of us (Serena) loves frozen peas and is writing this hack with her coauthor in mind when she says give "peas" a chance! Frozen peas are harvested at the peak of ripeness and are flash-frozen to maintain nutrition. They are rich in vitamins A, K, and C, and contain 5g protein and 4g fiber per ⅔-cup serving. The trick to liking frozen peas is to *not* cook them; simply thaw on the counter or add to hot water and immediately drain. Then toss them into salads, scrambled eggs, a can of soup, or any dish to which you want to add little pops of color, flavor, and nutrition.

Per Serving: Calories: 257; Total Fat: 10g; Saturated Fat: 2g; Cholesterol: 2mg; Sodium: 168mg; Total Carbohydrates: 37g; Fiber: 6g; Protein: 8g

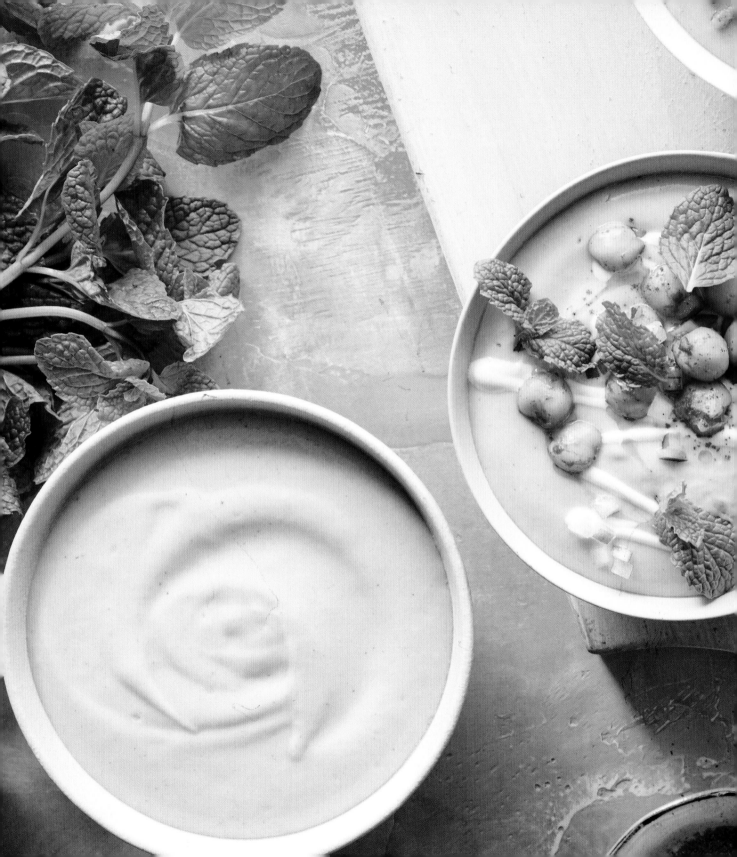

soups

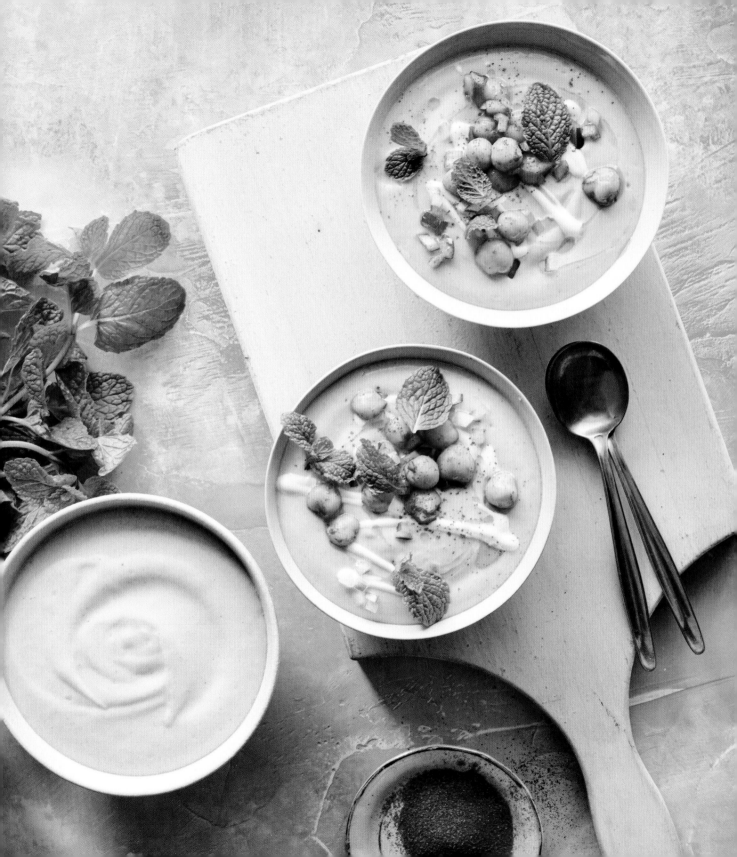

Cucumber-Avocado Gazpacho with Moroccan Chickpeas

Nut-Free, Gluten-Free, Egg-Free, Vegetarian	Serves 4	Prep time: 15 minutes

¼ cup plain 2% Greek yogurt

¼ cup mascarpone cheese or Neufchâtel cream cheese

1 avocado

1 lime

2 medium cucumbers, seeded and coarsely chopped (about 1¾ cups)

1 cup buttermilk

2 green onions

¼ cup plus 2 tablespoons fresh mint leaves, divided

¼ teaspoon kosher or sea salt

¼ teaspoon black pepper

1 (15-ounce) can chickpeas, drained and rinsed

¼ cup diced red onion

½ teaspoon smoked paprika

4 teaspoons extra-virgin olive oil

Deanna has never been a big fan of traditional gazpacho, the spicy Spanish tomato soup served cold. Then she tried this "green" version on a hot summer day, and she was hooked. The chickpeas add a decent amount of protein and fiber to make it a more substantial dish. Deanna likes to use mint here, but you could swap in fresh basil or cilantro instead.

In a small bowl, put the yogurt, mascarpone cheese, and 2 tablespoons water. Whip them together until smooth, adding another tablespoon or two of water, if needed, to create a drizzling consistency. Add half of the mixture to a blender and save the other half for garnishing the finished soup.

Cut the avocado in half and remove the pit with a spoon. Scoop the flesh into the blender. Squeeze 1 tablespoon of lime juice into the blender. (Save any remaining lime for another use.) Add the cucumbers, buttermilk, green onions, ¼ cup of the mint, the salt, and the black pepper. Blend until smooth. Chill the soup in the refrigerator until ready to serve.

In a medium bowl, mix the chickpeas, onion, and smoked paprika. Finely chop the remaining 2 tablespoons mint and add to the bowl. Mix well until the chickpeas are completely seasoned.

To serve, ladle the chilled soup into four bowls. Drizzle each bowl with the reserved yogurt mixture. Spoon the chickpeas on top of each serving. Drizzle each bowl with 1 teaspoon of the olive oil and serve.

Healthy Kitchen Hack: To make this soup vegan, swap in another avocado for the buttermilk, yogurt, and mascarpone cheese. Blend with the cucumbers, green onions, lime juice, salt, and pepper.

Per Serving: Calories: 344; Total Fat: 20g; Saturated Fat: 6g; Cholesterol: 28mg; Sodium: 443mg; Total Carbohydrates: 32g; Fiber: 9g; Protein: 11g

Savory Mushroom and Farro Soup

| Dairy-Free, Nut-Free, Egg-Free, Vegan | Serves 4 | Prep time: 5 minutes | Cook time: 30 minutes |

1 tablespoon extra-virgin olive oil

½ white or yellow onion, chopped (about 1 cup)

2 cups sliced baby bella mushrooms (8 ounces)

1 cup uncooked farro (6 ounces)

4 garlic cloves, minced

1 tablespoon fresh thyme or 1½ teaspoons dried

½ teaspoon kosher or sea salt

1 tablespoon red wine vinegar or white wine vinegar

Our Mediterranean spin on beef-and-barley soup might surprise you as the broth is so rich and filling, you may not believe it's just veggies and whole grains. The earthy mushrooms and the toasted farro are the secrets to the hearty, meaty flavor. Serena served this soup to a whole table of adults and kids who were unsure about farro, but their unanimous decision was that it might be even better than barley.

In a large stockpot over medium-high heat, heat the olive oil. Add the onion and cook for 5 minutes, stirring occasionally. Push the onion to the sides of the pot and add the mushrooms, then cook without stirring until a few of the mushrooms turn golden, 3 to 4 minutes. Push the mushrooms to the sides of the pot and add the farro, then cook without stirring until the farro toasts, 3 to 4 minutes. Add the garlic, thyme, and salt and cook, stirring frequently, for 1 minute. Add 5 cups water and stir. Increase the heat to high and bring the liquid to a boil. Once boiling, reduce the heat to medium-low, stir a few times, and cook until the farro is tender, 20 to 25 minutes. Stir in the vinegar and serve.

Healthy Kitchen Hack: Farro might become your new favorite way to add plant-based protein to your meals. While quinoa is known as a protein-rich whole grain with 6 grams of protein per serving, farro actually has 7 grams of protein along with 5 grams of fiber. To enrich your meals with farro, add cooked farro to pancakes, muffins, and banana bread. Stir it into homemade or canned soups. Use it as a base for grain bowls as we do in the Spiced Carrot-Hummus Bowls (page 207) or in place of rice on your dinner plate.

Per Serving: Calories: 234; Total Fat: 5g; Saturated Fat: 1g; Cholesterol: 0mg; Sodium: 245mg; Total Carbohydrates: 42g; Fiber: 6g; Protein: 9g

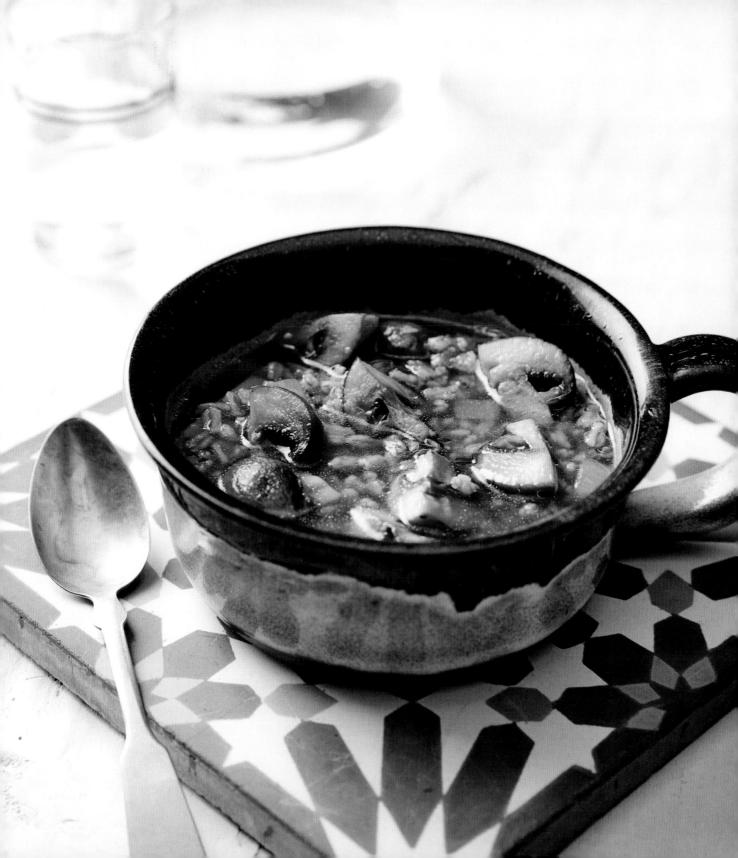

Mediterranean Lentil Chili

Nut-Free, Gluten-Free, Egg-Free, Vegetarian	Serves 8	Prep time: 5 minutes	Cook time: 30 minutes

1 tablespoon extra-virgin olive oil

1 medium onion, diced

1 large bell pepper (any color), seeded and chopped

1 small jalapeño pepper, seeded and chopped

2 garlic cloves, minced

2 teaspoons ground cumin

2 teaspoons smoked paprika

3 cups low-sodium or no-salt-added vegetable broth

1 (28-ounce) can no-salt-added diced tomatoes

1 (15-ounce) can pinto beans, drained and rinsed

¾ cup uncooked brown or green lentils, rinsed

½ cup plain 2% Greek yogurt (about 4 ounces)

1 cup shredded cheese like Monterey Jack, Colby Jack, or cheddar (about 4 ounces)

This meatless chili features lentils—a Mediterranean staple legume that we love to use in recipes because they cook up fairly quickly and are loaded with protein and fiber. Any leftovers taste even better the next day after the ingredients have time to concentrate and meld together while sitting in your refrigerator. If you have fresh cilantro, parsley, or chives on hand, chop them up to use as a topping, or try adding the surprise ingredient we feature in our Healthy Kitchen Hack below.

In a large stockpot, heat the olive oil over medium heat. Add the onion, bell pepper, and jalapeño. Cook, stirring frequently, until slightly softened, about 5 minutes. Add the garlic, cumin, and smoked paprika. Cook, stirring frequently, for 30 seconds. Add the broth, tomatoes, pinto beans, and lentils. Bring to a boil, then reduce the heat to medium-low. Cover the pot with a lid and cook until the lentils have softened, 20 to 25 minutes.

To serve, ladle the chili into bowls and top with the yogurt and shredded cheese.

Healthy Kitchen Hack: Whenever you have extra canned pumpkin or leftovers of our Roasted Butternut Squash (page 77), add them to this chili! Simply mix into the pot after the lentils have cooked and heat for an additional 10 minutes. You won't even taste it, but you'll get some extra veggie vitamins and minerals in your chili bowl; plus, it will make your chili extra-thick.

Per Serving: Calories: 264; Total Fat: 7g; Saturated Fat: 3g; Cholesterol: 15mg; Sodium: 365mg; Total Carbohydrates: 35g; Fiber: 8g; Protein: 16g

Creamy Chickpea-Tahini Soup

Dairy-Free, Nut-Free, Gluten-Free, Egg-Free, Vegan	Serves 6	Prep time: 10 minutes	Cook time: 30 minutes

1 tablespoon extra-virgin olive oil

½ small white or yellow onion, chopped

3 celery stalks, chopped

3 garlic cloves, minced

1 teaspoon dried thyme

½ teaspoon kosher or sea salt

¼ teaspoon black pepper

4 cups low-sodium or no-salt-added vegetable broth

2 (15-ounce) cans chickpeas, drained and rinsed, divided

3 tablespoons tahini

1 medium lemon, cut in half

⅓ cup chopped fresh cilantro leaves and stems

1 tablespoon sesame seeds

If you are a hummus lover, we think you'll become an instant fan of this vegan soup. Pureeing cooked beans is clever way to thicken your broth while mimicking the silky texture of a creamed soup without using milk. If you don't have to avoid dairy, though, swirl a dollop of plain Greek yogurt into your blended soup for an extra-smooth and velvety consistency.

In a large stockpot over medium heat, heat the olive oil. Add the onion, celery, garlic, thyme, salt, and black pepper and stir well. Reduce the heat to medium-low and cook, stirring occasionally, until the vegetables have softened, about 10 minutes.

Add the broth and 1½ cans of the chickpeas, then increase the heat to medium-high. Bring the soup to a boil, then reduce the heat to medium. Simmer until the chickpeas are very soft, about 15 minutes. Remove from the heat.

Carefully ladle half of the hot soup into a blender, leaving an opening at the top covered with a clean towel to prevent a buildup of steam, and puree until smooth. (For best results, use a standing blender instead of an immersion blender to get the desired velvety texture.) Pour the blended soup into a large bowl and repeat with the remaining soup. Return the pureed soup to the pot. Add the tahini and whisk. Squeeze 1 teaspoon of lemon juice into the pot. (Save any remaining lemon for another use.) Add the remaining ½ can chickpeas, stir, and cook for 2 to 3 minutes until heated through. Ladle the soup into bowls and top with the cilantro and sesame seeds.

continued

Creamy Chickpea-Tahini Soup (continued)

Healthy Kitchen Hack: Deanna has created the ultimate shortcut to making a similar version this soup using only two ingredients! In a medium saucepan, whisk together a 10-ounce tub of prepared hummus with 1 cup low-sodium or no-salt-added vegetable broth. Warm over medium heat until ready to serve. Makes 2 servings. (Note: The nutrition analysis will be different than listed below.)

Per Serving: Calories: 251; Total Fat: 10g; Saturated Fat: 1g; Cholesterol: 0mg; Sodium: 596mg; Total Carbohydrates: 32g; Fiber: 10g; Protein: 10g

"WOW! This recipe sounded strange at first, but it was so much better than I expected. I even had two bowls the next day . . . for breakfast!"

—Bonnie from Lakewood, CO

Yiayia's Avgolemono Lemon Chicken Soup

Dairy-Free, Nut-Free	Serves 6	Prep time: 10 minutes	Cook time: 20 minutes

1 boneless, skinless chicken breast (8 to 10 ounces)

1 teaspoon kosher or sea salt

½ teaspoon black pepper

8 ounces uncooked orzo pasta

4 large eggs

2 medium lemons, cut in half

Serena's friend John speaks seven languages, including Greek. As a teenager, he learned to make this thick, rich chicken soup from his friend's Greek *yiayia* (grandmother). She taught John an avgolemono (or egg-lemon) soup recipe that traditionally took two days to make! He then shared it with Serena, along with the simple technique of how to add eggs to the hot broth so they don't curdle. The trick works perfectly in this soup recipe, too—but this one takes only about 30 minutes. And it still tastes just as *nostimo* (*NOH-stee-mo*)—Greek for "delicious"!

Into a large stockpot, put 7 cups water and the chicken breast, salt, and black pepper. Bring to a boil over medium-high heat. Stir in the orzo. Cook, stirring occasionally, until the orzo is tender but still al dente and the internal temperature of the chicken measures 165°F on a meat thermometer, about 10 minutes. Turn the heat off.

While the chicken and orzo cook, crack the eggs into a medium bowl. Squeeze ¼ cup of lemon juice into the bowl. (Save any remaining lemon for another use.) Whisk until smooth and set aside.

Using a slotted spoon, remove the chicken to a plate or cutting board and carefully shred the meat using two forks. Add the chicken back to the soup along with ½ cup cold water. Check the temperature of the soup with a meat thermometer: It should be 165° to 180°F in order to be cool enough to add the eggs without them curdling. (If it's hotter than 180°F, stir the soup a bit to lower the temperature.)

While whisking constantly, ladle ½ cup of the hot broth into the bowl with the egg mixture. Then, while whisking constantly, add the egg mixture to the soup in the pot in a very small, slow stream. Turn the heat back on to low and cook, stirring constantly, until the soup becomes opaque and thickens, 1 to 2 minutes.

continued

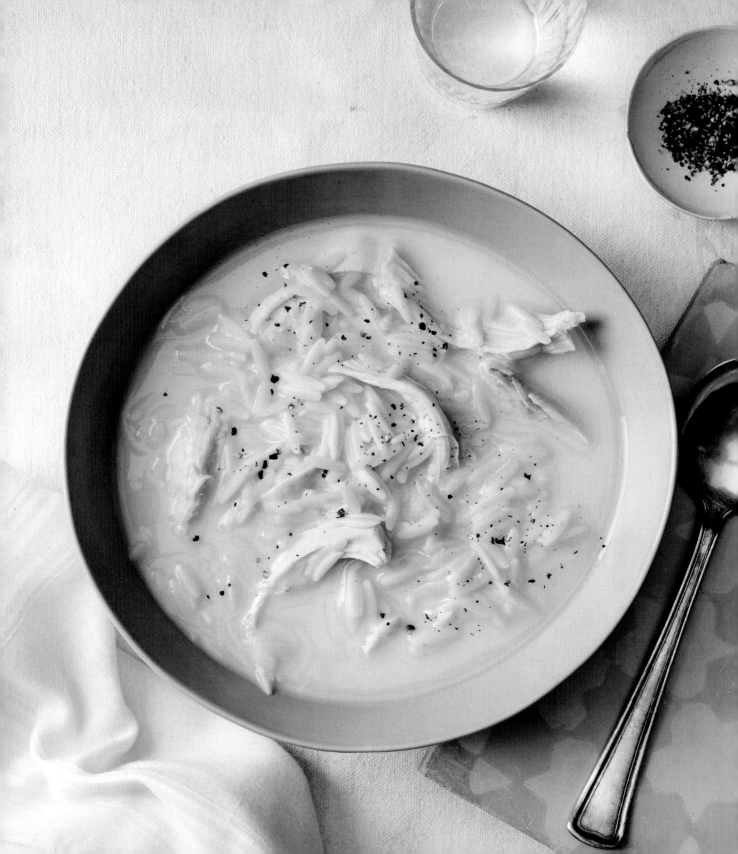

Healthy Kitchen Hack: To get more whole grains on your table, use instant brown rice instead of orzo. Make the soup as described, except add 2 cups uncooked instant brown rice to the pot with the water, chicken, salt, and black pepper before turning on the heat. Once the pot boils, cook for 10 minutes, turn the heat off, and follow the rest of the recipe directions.

Per Serving: Calories: 248; Total Fat: 5g; Cholesterol: 159mg; Sodium: 391 mg; Total Carbohydrates: 30g; Fiber: 1g; Protein: 20g

"I heartily approve this version! Yiayia's recipe didn't have big chunks of meaty chicken in it, but I really like that addition."

—John from Edwardsville, IL

Monday Minestrone Soup

Nut-Free, Egg-free, Vegetarian	Serves 6	Prep time: 10 minutes	Cook time: 20 minutes

1 tablespoon extra-virgin olive oil

1 medium onion, chopped

2 carrots, chopped

2 celery stalks, chopped

3 garlic cloves, minced

¾ teaspoon dried thyme

8 cups low-sodium vegetable broth

1 (28-ounce) can low-sodium diced tomatoes

½ (16-ounce) bag or 1 (10-ounce) box frozen spinach

8 ounces uncooked whole-grain or regular elbow pasta

1 (15-ounce) can cannellini beans, drained and rinsed

¼ teaspoon kosher or sea salt

¼ teaspoon black pepper

½ cup plus 1 tablespoon grated Parmesan or Pecorino Romano cheese

This vegetarian (or vegan if you hold the cheese) is a win-win-win. It's a breeze to make; is loaded with plant-based protein, fiber, vitamins, and minerals; and is a super-satisfying one-pot meal. Deanna recommends making a big batch of it on Sunday, so you don't even have to think about what's for dinner on Monday—simply reheat and serve!

In a large stockpot, heat the olive oil over medium heat. Add the onion, carrots, celery, and garlic. Cook, stirring occasionally, until the vegetables soften, about 10 minutes. Add the thyme and stir frequently for 30 seconds. Add the broth and tomatoes and bring to a boil over high heat.

Once boiling, add the frozen spinach (no need to thaw) and wait for the soup to start boiling again. Add the pasta, reduce the heat to medium-high, and stir. Cook for the amount of time recommended on the box of pasta for al dente, stirring occasionally.

Once the pasta is cooked, add the beans, salt, and black pepper. Stir and reduce the heat to medium. Cook for another few minutes until the beans are warm. Ladle the soup into bowls and top each with 1½ tablespoons of the grated cheese.

Healthy Kitchen Hack: Give this vegetarian soup another huge flavor boost with roasted garlic. If you have the time, it's worth letting your oven transform a head of raw garlic into silky, smooth, and mellow garlic paste. Remove the outer papery layers but keep the cloves attached to the head. Cut off the tops of the cloves and place the head on a piece of aluminum foil. Drizzle the top of the garlic with a teaspoon of olive oil and close the foil loosely around the head. Roast in a 400°F oven for at least 45 minutes until the cloves have completely softened. Cool slightly, then squeeze out all the cloves (yes, all of them as they are mild compared to raw garlic) and use in recipes by stirring into the pan when you would usually add raw garlic. You can also mix roasted garlic into dips, use it as a sandwich spread, or whisk it into dressings.

Per Serving: Calories: 357; Total Fat: 6g; Saturated Fat: 2g; Cholesterol: 5mg; Sodium: 732mg; Total Carbohydrates: 61g; Fiber: 12g; Protein: 18g

"This was super delicious—I ate it for three days straight! I added crushed red pepper and more black pepper for an extra kick."

—Robin from Dallas, TX

Italian Wedding Soup with Meatballs

Nut-Free, Egg-Free, Vegetarian | **Serves 6** | Prep time: 10 minutes | Cook time: 25 minutes

4 cups low-sodium or no-salt-added vegetable broth

2 (2-inch) pieces Parmesan cheese rinds or any hard cheese

1 tablespoon extra-virgin olive oil

½ medium onion, chopped (about 1 cup)

4 garlic cloves, minced

1 tablespoon dried oregano

½ teaspoon kosher or sea salt

¼ teaspoon black pepper

2 tablespoons tomato paste

1 bunch kale, leaves stemmed and torn into bite-size pieces (about 6 cups)

8 ounces uncooked orzo pasta

16 cooked meatballs like Chickpea "Meatballs" (page 217) or Best Baked Italian Meatballs (page 230)

1 tablespoon white wine vinegar or red wine vinegar

Choose your meatball "path" to this hearty soup: one road leads to our veggie-loaded Chickpea "Meatballs" and the other yummy option is our Best Baked Italian Meatballs. Either choice leads to a delicious bowl of classic comfort food with a Mediterranean twist that can include options of what's currently in your fridge or freezer. Don't have kale? Use cabbage instead (we tested it, it's delish). Got a few extra fresh herbs? Throw them in, too. No time to make meatballs or none in the freezer? Swap in a can of beans instead.

Put the broth and cheese rinds in a medium saucepan and heat over medium heat. Let the cheese steep while you prepare the rest of the soup.

In a large stockpot over medium-high heat, heat the olive oil. Add the onion and cook, stirring occasionally, for 5 minutes. Add the garlic, oregano, salt, and black pepper and cook, stirring frequently, for 1 minute. Add 8 cups water, the tomato paste, and the warm cheese broth to the stockpot. Stir and bring to a boil over high heat. Add the kale and orzo. Stir a few times, reduce the heat to medium-high, and cook at a simmer until the pasta is cooked, stirring occasionally, 12 to 15 minutes. Reduce the heat to medium and add the meatballs; cook until the meatballs are heated through. Using a slotted spoon, remove the cheese rinds. Add the vinegar, stir, and serve.

Healthy Kitchen Hack: We encourage you to buy blocks of aged cheese versus grated or shredded Parmesan or Pecorino Romano. Your cheese will stay fresher longer (wrap it in parchment paper, not plastic wrap, so it can breathe!), and you get the bonus of the rinds—rich, savory flavor bombs. Freeze the rinds for when you make a stew or soup like this one and toss them in straight from the freezer. You can also buy "Parmesan ends" at the supermarket deli or at a cheese shop, which is a budget-friendly way to enjoy pricier aged cheeses.

Per Serving (with Chickpea "Meatballs"): Calories: 375; Total Fat: 9g; Saturated Fat: 1.5g; Cholesterol: 5mg; Sodium: 830mg; Total Carbohydrates: 57g; Fiber: 10g; Protein: 16g

"I can't believe the broth was my favorite part of this recipe. The Chickpea 'Meatballs' were really good and so was the whole soup, but the broth with oregano, onion, garlic, and cheese rinds was so flavorful!"

—Dale from Delta, PA

Pork, Apple, and Butternut Squash Stew with Sage

Nut-Free, Gluten-Free, Egg-Free	Serves 6	Prep time: 15 minutes	Cook time: 35 minutes

1½ pounds boneless pork loin

1 medium lemon, cut in half

2 tablespoons extra-virgin olive oil, divided

2 garlic cloves, minced

1 tablespoon plus 1 teaspoon chopped fresh sage leaves or rosemary or 1½ teaspoons dried, divided

1 medium white or yellow onion

¼ cup dry white wine

2 cups low-sodium or no-salt-added chicken broth

2 tablespoons tomato paste

1 (2- to 3-pound) butternut squash or 2 (10-ounce) packages frozen cubed squash

2 medium apples, any variety, chopped

1 tablespoon dried oregano

½ teaspoon black pepper

¼ teaspoon kosher or sea salt

½ cup (2 ounces) crumbled blue cheese

While writing this book, the Ball family got a visit from Eric, a good friend who works as an archaeologist in Cyprus. This simple stew was inspired by the flavors of Cypriot food interwoven in his stories. Eric described excavating a 5,000-year-old city from beneath a modern-day orchard, being cautious of the apple tree roots as he dug. The family who owned the orchard cooked many apple dishes, some like this. Additionally, sage is native to the Mediterranean region, including Cyprus, where it's used in meat dishes along with seasonal vegetables and black pepper.

Trim the fat from all the edges of the pork and discard. Slice the pork into 1-inch cubes and pat them dry with a paper towel.

Squeeze 2 tablespoons of lemon juice into a large glass bowl. (Save any remaining lemon for another use.) Add the pork, 1 tablespoon of the olive oil, the garlic, and 1 teaspoon of the fresh sage (or ½ teaspoon dried). Cover and marinate on the counter while you prep the veggies, at least 10 minutes.

While the pork marinates, on a clean cutting board, slice the onion in half from sprout to root end. Peel and slice into thin half-moon slices.

Peel the butternut squash and cut it into ¾-inch cubes. (For peeling tips, see the Healthy Kitchen Hack on page 79.)

In a large stockpot over medium-high heat, heat the remaining 1 tablespoon olive oil for at least 3 minutes until very hot. Add the pork to the pot so as many pieces as possible touch the hot oil. Top the pork with the onions, but do not stir the pork until it browns, about 4 minutes. Add the wine and stir well, scraping up any browned bits on the bottom of the pot. Cook until most of the wine has evaporated, about 2 minutes. Stir in the broth, tomato paste, squash, apples, and 1 cup water. Add the remaining 1 tablespoon sage and the oregano, black pepper, and salt. Bring to a boil. Reduce the heat to low and simmer, uncovered, until the squash has softened, about 20 minutes.

Place the blue cheese in a small serving bowl to serve alongside the stew.

Healthy Kitchen Hack: When you need wine for a recipe, avoid "cooking wines" (added salt!) and choose a wine you'd likely drink with that dish. When a recipe calls for dry red wine, options include Merlot, Pinot Noir, lighter Cabernets, and Sangiovese. Some good dry white wines are Chenin Blanc, Viognier, Chardonnay, Pinot Gris, and Sauvignon Blanc.

Per Serving: Calories: 342; **Total Fat:** 12g; **Saturated Fat:** 4g; **Cholesterol:** 79mg; **Sodium:** 293mg; **Total Carbohydrates:** 30g; **Fiber:** 4g; **Protein:** 31g

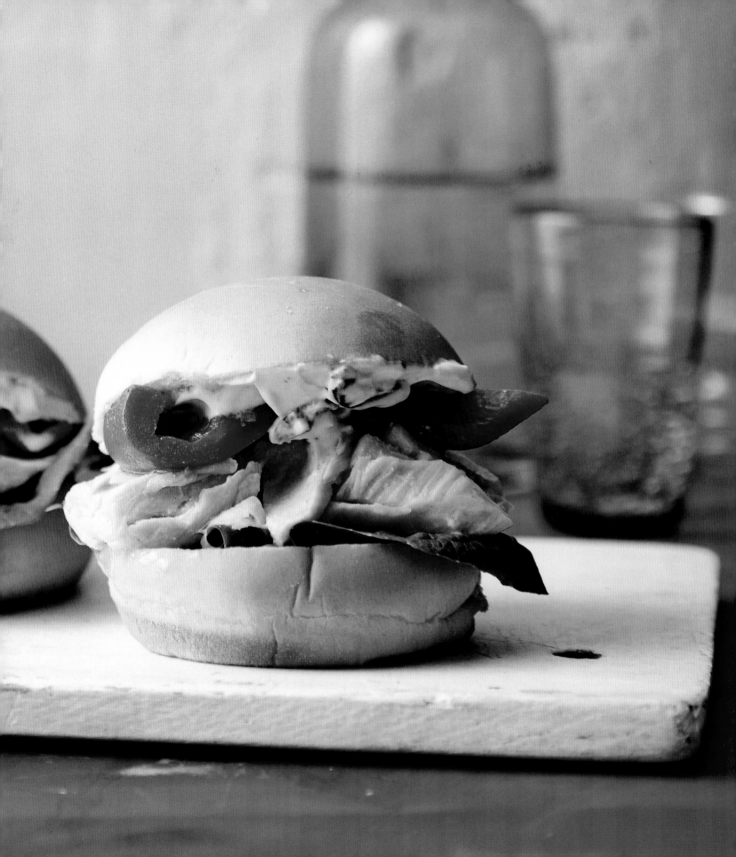

sandwiches

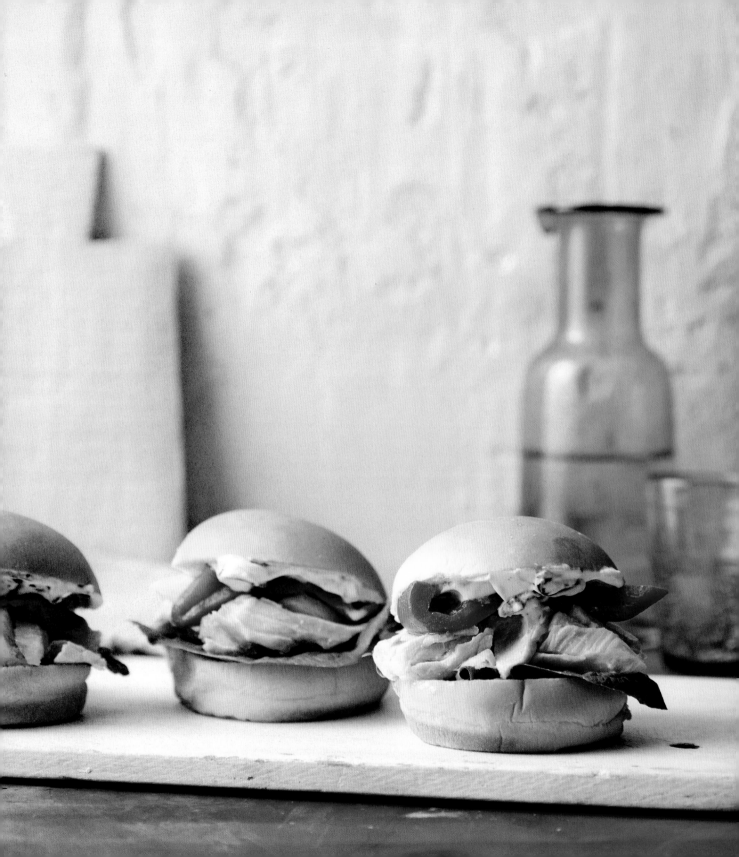

Salmon Sliders with Kalamata Olive-Yogurt Sauce

| Nut-Free, Egg-Free | Serves 4 | Prep time: 10 minutes | Cook time: 5 minutes |

1 pound skinless salmon, cut into 4 pieces

¼ teaspoon black pepper

½ cup plain (2%) Greek yogurt

⅓ cup chopped pitted Kalamata olives, 2 tablespoons of liquid from the jar reserved

8 mini whole-grain hamburger buns or other slider buns, split

1 roasted red pepper (from a 12-ounce jar or homemade—see page 44), cut into 8 pieces

2 romaine lettuce leaves, each cut into 4 pieces

These sliders were inspired by the time Deanna had a deadline to develop a fish recipe, but the gas line to her house (and stove!) was turned off. By using her microwave and some Mediterranean-style pantry staples, she was able to whip up these yummy olive and salmon mini-sandwiches in minutes. Since then, both she and a few of our fans have tested them to perfection.

Put the salmon fillets in a glass pie plate. Sprinkle with the black pepper. Cover the dish with plastic wrap, leaving a small part open at the edge to vent the steam. Microwave on high power for about 3 minutes. The fish is done when it just begins to separate into flakes (chunks) when pressed gently with a fork. Divide into 8 portions.

While the fish cooks, in a small bowl, whisk together the yogurt, olives, and olive liquid.

To assemble sliders, place one portion of the salmon on each bottom bun. Top each with two roasted pepper pieces. Spread the olive yogurt sauce over the peppers. Top each slider with 2 pieces of lettuce and the bun tops.

Healthy Kitchen Hack: Save that olive juice! Whether it's brine from a jar of Kalamata olives or the mild liquid from canned green olives, the juice adds instant flavor and appeal to so many condiments. Mix a few tablespoons into salad dressing or even plain yogurt for a dip, sandwich spread, or vegetable topper like in our Greek Zucchini Pita Nachos on page 197.

Per Serving: Calories: 468; Total Fat: 11g; Saturated Fat: 3g; Cholesterol: 62mg; Sodium: 1,088 mg; Total Carbohydrates: 51g; Fiber: 7g; Protein: 28g

"Microwaving the salmon was my favorite part of this recipe—I love how the fish gets perfectly cooked. This meal was speedy enough to make after work and before a night meeting."

—Kate from Hamel, IL

Rosemary-Roasted Pork and Provolone Sandwiches

Nut-Free, Egg-Free	Serves 6	Prep time: 10 minutes	Cook time: 15 minutes

1 tablespoon chopped fresh
rosemary leaves

¼ teaspoon garlic powder

1 pork tenderloin (about
1 pound), cut in half crosswise

2 tablespoons extra-olive oil,
divided

½ teaspoon kosher or sea salt

1 bunch broccoli rabe (about
12 ounces), cut into 1-inch
pieces

2 garlic cloves, minced

⅛ teaspoon crushed red
pepper

1 (12-ounce) baguette

3 ounces sliced provolone
cheese

2 roasted red peppers (from
a 12-ounce jar or homemade—
see page 44), drained and
sliced

If you ask Deanna where to get a Philly cheesesteak in her hometown of Philadelphia, she'll instead encourage you to order the locals' real favorite sandwich: slow-roasted pork with sharp provolone and spicy broccoli rabe. While this specific sandwich is a Philly favorite, the fillings are all staple ingredients in the Mediterranean Diet, so we had to share it here. Deanna includes roasted red peppers in her version for a touch of sweetness, a kick of color, and an extra serving of veggies.

Preheat the oven to 450°F.

In a small bowl, mix together the rosemary and garlic powder, then rub all over both pieces of the pork tenderloin.

Pour 1 tablespoon of the olive oil into a large ovenproof skillet and heat over medium-high heat. Add the tenderloin halves and sear for 1 minute. Using tongs, turn the pieces over and sear for another minute. Transfer the skillet to the oven and roast the pork for 5 minutes, then, using tongs, turn both pieces over. Cook for an additional 5 to 8 minutes or until the internal temperature of each piece measures 145°F on a meat thermometer. Remove the skillet from the oven and place the pork on a cutting board. Let it rest for 5 minutes and then slice thinly.

While the pork is cooking, bring a large stockpot of water to a boil. Add the salt and broccoli rabe, and cook for 2 minutes. Drain.

Return the empty stockpot to the stove and turn the heat to medium. Add the remaining 1 tablespoon olive oil and heat for about 15 seconds. Add the garlic and crushed red pepper; cook, stirring frequently, for 30 seconds. Add the broccoli rabe and cook, stirring occasionally, until tender but not mushy, 6 to 8 minutes. Remove from the heat.

continued

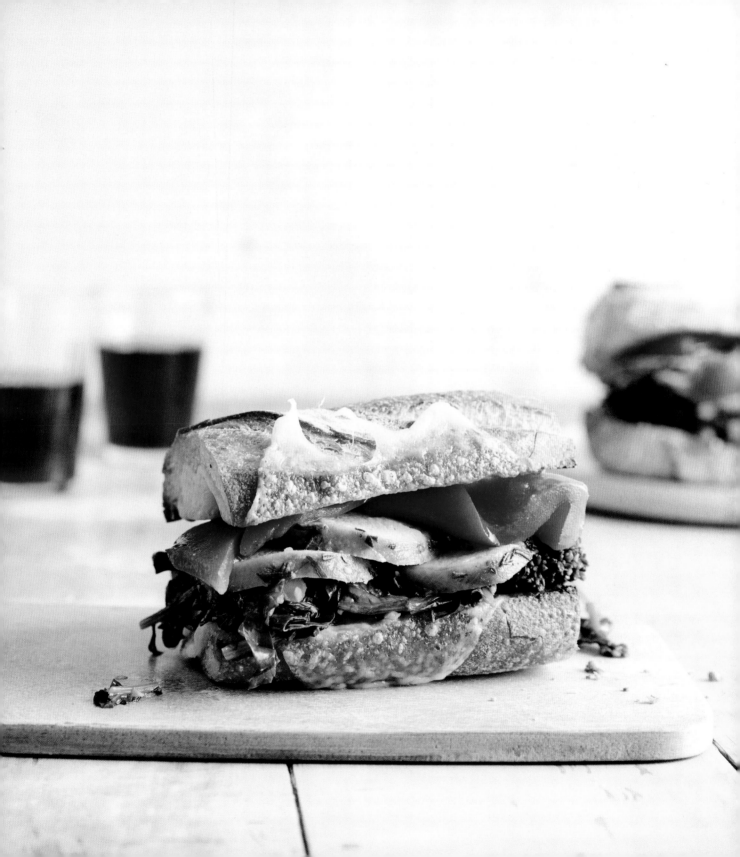

Turn the broiler to high.

Cut the baguette crosswise into six pieces. Cut each piece lengthwise almost all the way through so it resembles a small sub roll. Open up each sub roll (still keeping the bread connected) and place on a large rimmed baking sheet, cut-side up. Add the cheese on one side of each roll. Broil until the bread is toasted and the cheese is melted, 1½ to 2 minutes.

To assemble, divide the sliced pork evenly among the six rolls. Top with the broccoli rabe and roasted peppers.

Healthy Kitchen Hack: Also known as rapini, broccoli rabe is a member of the cruciferous family, which includes vegetables like broccoli, cauliflower, and cabbage. While it's loaded with nutrients like vitamins A, C, and K, folate, and fiber, it can taste bitter. A quick boil in salted water is the secret to help tamp down the bitterness. To serve broccoli rabe as a side, sauté it with garlic and crushed red pepper along with a few chopped anchovies. Also, toss broccoli rabe with pasta or roasted potatoes for a delectable combination.

Per Serving: Calories: 337; Total Fat: 10g; Saturated Fat: 4g; Cholesterol: 59mg; Sodium: 626mg; Total Carbohydrates: 35g; Fiber: 3g; Protein: 21g

"The pork was perfectly cooked, tender and juicy. This was my first time making broccoli rabe, and with the peppers, it made for a pretty appealing sandwich!"

—Emily from Worthington, OH

E.A.L.T. (Egg Avocado Lettuce Tomato) Wraps

| Vegetarian | Serves 4 | Prep time: 10 minutes | Cook time: 5 minutes |

1 tablespoon extra-virgin olive oil

4 large eggs

4 teaspoons pesto, homemade (see page 153) or store-bought

4 whole-wheat wraps

4 romaine lettuce leaves

1 avocado, pitted, peeled, and sliced

1 small tomato, sliced

½ teaspoon smoked paprika

"These were delicious! I loved the creaminess of the egg and avocado mixed with the crunchy lettuce and juicy tomato along with the heat of the smoked paprika. My husband and (not-so-adventurous) 8-year-old daughter loved them, too."

—Sheila from Baltimore, MD

For our meat-free Mediterranean twist on the classic BLT, we feature the almond pesto from our Penne with Almond Pesto and Eggplant recipe as the sandwich spread. We also add a few shakes of Deanna's favorite spice, smoked paprika, to jazz up the egg and replace the smokiness the bacon lends a traditional BLT. Feel free to switch up the sandwich bread to pita pockets or slices of toasted Italian bread.

Heat a large skillet over medium heat and pour in the olive oil. Gently crack the eggs into the skillet. Cook until the egg whites are opaque, 2 minutes. Flip each egg and cook until the yolks are set, 1 to 2 minutes. Remove the eggs from the pan to a plate.

To assemble the wraps, spread 1 teaspoon of the pesto over each wrap. Add a lettuce leaf on top followed by avocado slices. Add the tomato slices and top with one fried egg. Sprinkle each egg with ⅛ teaspoon of the of smoked paprika. Fold up the bottom about 2 inches. Fold the left side over, covering the fillings, then fold the right side over that, and serve.

Healthy Kitchen Hack: Made from smoke-dried pimento peppers, smoked paprika is a tantalizing spice that can provide the smoky, meaty flavor of bacon, prosciutto, or chorizo to vegetarian or vegan recipes without the use of meat. A staple in Spanish dishes, smoked paprika is most commonly used in paella, meat marinades, and barbecue rubs, but Deanna adds it to just about any savory dish that needs a warm and smoky—but not too spicy—kick.

Per Serving: Calories: 317; Total Fat: 20g; Saturated Fat: 5g; Cholesterol: 186mg; Sodium: 338mg; Total Carbohydrates: 24g; Fiber: 7g; Protein: 12g

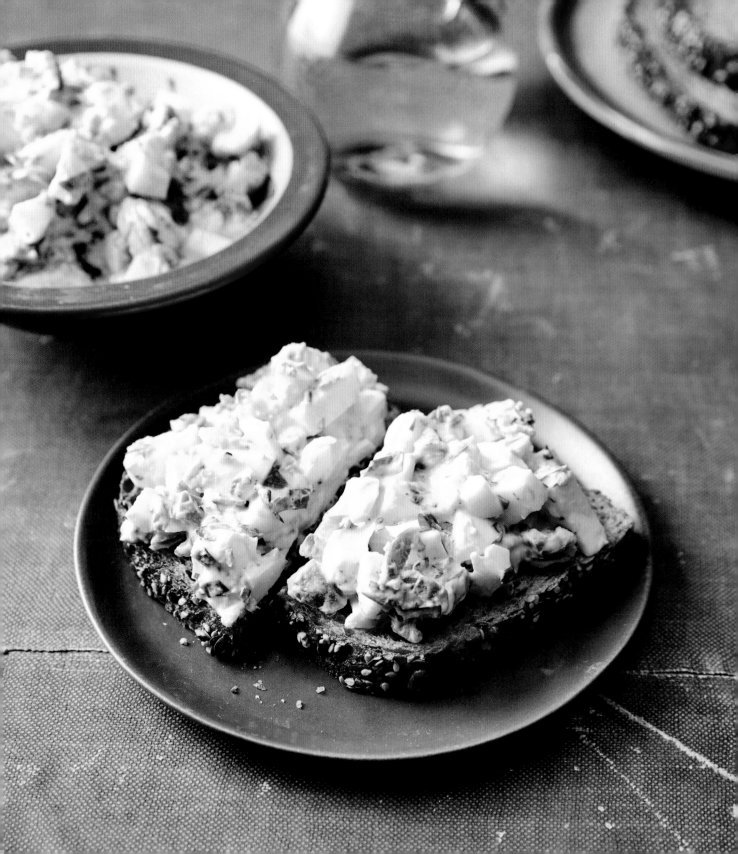

Olive Egg Salad Sandwiches

| Nut-Free, Vegetarian | Serves 4 | Prep time: 10 minutes | Cook time: 15 minutes |

½ cup plain 2% Greek yogurt (about 4 ounces)

1 tablespoon extra-virgin olive oil

½ teaspoon black pepper

⅛ teaspoon kosher or sea salt

5 hard-boiled large eggs, peeled and chopped (see Healthy Kitchen Hack below)

½ cup chopped fresh parsley

¼ cup chopped pitted green olives

4 slices crusty whole-grain bread

The first time Serena had an egg-salad-and-green-olive combo, she was vacationing in sunny Florida. When she re-created it back home in her own kitchen, she tested it with our Olive Oil–Yogurt Spread (page 42) instead of the typical mayonnaise, to delicious results. For this open-face sandwich, feel free to swap in your favorite fresh green herb for the parsley. Serena likes to use fresh dill and will go as far as adding one full cup of it; after all, the Mediterranean way is to use cups of herbs, instead of tablespoons.

In a medium bowl, whisk together the yogurt, olive oil, black pepper, and salt. Add the eggs, parsley, and olives. Stir until all the ingredients are mixed together.

Toast the bread slices in the toaster or warm in a 200°F oven for 5 minutes until toasted. Divide the egg salad among the toasts and serve.

Healthy Kitchen Hack: Yes, you can make hard-cooked eggs that are a breeze to peel, perfectly cooked, and without the green tinge around the yolk. (The green ring is perfectly fine to eat; it's just a reaction from the egg being overboiled.) Instead of boiling, consider steaming your eggs. (They will be easier to peel!) Place a large pot with 1 inch of water over high heat. Cover and bring to a boil. Once boiling, remove the lid and place a steamer basket or metal colander over the boiling water. Add 5 large eggs to the steamer and cover again. Steam for 10½ to 11 minutes. Using oven mitts, immediately remove the steamer from the pot and carefully place the eggs in a large bowl of ice water to cool.

Per Serving: Calories: 281; Total Fat: 14g; Saturated Fat: 3g; Cholesterol: 235mg; Sodium: 384mg; Total Carbohydrates: 26g; Fiber: 3g; Protein: 15g

Middle Eastern Chicken Schnitzel Sandwich

| Dairy-Free, Nut-Free | Serves 4 | Prep time: 15 minutes | Cook time: 10 minutes |

1 pound boneless, skinless chicken breasts

2 tablespoons cornmeal

1 large egg

⅔ cup panko breadcrumbs

2 tablespoons sesame seeds

2 garlic cloves, minced

¼ teaspoon black pepper

½ teaspoon kosher or sea salt, divided

1 tablespoon extra-virgin olive oil

1½ cups sliced cucumber (about 1 English seedless cucumber)

2 tablespoons white wine vinegar or rice vinegar

⅛ teaspoon crushed red pepper

1½ tablespoons tahini

1½ teaspoons honey

4 whole-wheat hot dog buns

1 medium lemon, cut in half

Originating in Austria, many versions of schnitzel have been adopted by countries around the globe, including Israel. Chicken schnitzel is a favorite comfort food often offered sandwich style, much like falafel in quick-serve restaurants called *shuks* and street carts throughout the country. Along with pita, bun-style bread is an option, served with hummus, pickles, ketchup, or spicy mayo as condiments. Here we opt for a sesame-panko breading for the chicken served on whole-grain hot dog buns (to accommodate the long pieces of chicken) with pickled cucumbers and honey-tahini sauce as the extras.

Place the chicken between two pieces of plastic wrap. Using a meat mallet, metal ladle, or a small frying pan, pound the chicken to a ¼-inch thickness. Remove the breasts from the plastic wrap and cut into four pieces total. Set aside.

Measure the cornmeal into a large bowl. Into another large bowl, crack the egg and add 1 tablespoon water; whisk together. In a third large bowl, mix together the panko, sesame seeds, garlic, and black pepper.

Pat dry the chicken pieces with a paper towel and sprinkle each with ¼ teaspoon of the salt. Dip one piece in the cornmeal mixture and turn to make sure both sides are fully covered. Next, dip the chicken into the egg mixture to coat it on both sides. Slide any excess back into the bowl with your hands. Last, dip the egg-covered chicken into the panko coating, turning to make sure both sides are fully covered. Place the coated chicken on a plate and repeat the coating process with the remaining chicken pieces.

In a large skillet, heat the olive oil over medium heat. Add the chicken pieces and cook for 4 minutes. Flip each piece and cook until a meat thermometer inserted into the chicken registers 165°F, 3 to 4 more minutes.

While the chicken is cooking, in a large bowl, put the cucumber, vinegar, remaining ¼ teaspoon salt, and the crushed red pepper. Combine well and set aside.

In another small bowl, put the tahini, honey, and 1 tablespoon water. Whisk well and set aside.

To assemble the sandwiches, spread the tahini sauce on one half of each hot dog bun. Add the chicken schnitzel and a squeeze of juice from one lemon half (save the other lemon half for another use). Top with the cucumber mixture and serve.

Healthy Kitchen Hack: For even more yummy (and healthy!) condiment ideas for your schnitzel sandwich, check out the options we give for our Grilled Veggie Gyros (page 124), Falafel Wraps (page 120), and Turkey Shawarma (page 259).

Per Serving: Calories: 454; Total Fat: 15g; Saturated Fat: 2g; Cholesterol: 129mg; Sodium: 563mg; Total Carbohydrates: 44g; Fiber: 4g; Protein: 36g

Falafel Wraps with Lemon Yogurt-Tahini Spread

Egg-Free, Vegetarian	Serves 4	Prep time: 20 minutes	Cook time: 15 minutes

1 (15-ounce) can chickpeas, drained and rinsed, liquid reserved

2 cups chopped fresh parsley, divided

2 tablespoons white whole-wheat flour

2 tablespoons tahini or peanut butter, divided

1 garlic clove

2 teaspoons ground cumin

¼ teaspoon crushed red pepper (optional)

¼ teaspoon kosher or sea salt

2 tablespoons plus 1 teaspoon extra-virgin olive oil, divided

1 medium lemon, cut in half

½ cup plain 2% Greek yogurt (4 ounces)

4 whole-wheat flatbread wraps or soft whole-wheat tortillas

1 medium tomato, sliced

The hardest part of making this sandwich might be deciding which condiment to use on it! The citrusy, tart, creamy, and nutty sauce we use here is superb—but so is our Olive Oil–Yogurt Spread (page 42), as is the tzatziki sauce from the Grilled Veggie Gyros (page 124). In fact, when Serena was making these wraps, she tried them *all*. In the end, this sauce made the cut for this wrap because some of these ingredients were already in the crispy, crunchy chickpea falafel patties. But feel free to mix and match all our options to make a unique sandwich every time.

Place a large rimmed baking sheet on the middle rack in the oven. Preheat the oven to 400°F.

Into a food processor, put the chickpeas, 1 tablespoon of the reserved chickpea liquid, 1 cup of the parsley, the flour, 1 tablespoon of the tahini, garlic, the cumin, crushed red pepper, and salt. Pulse about 10 times until the mixture is combined (but not pureed); add 1 to 2 tablespoons more chickpea liquid if needed until the mixture comes together. Using a 1½-tablespoon scoop, make 12 falafel patties and place on a plate.

Remove the hot baking sheet from the oven and pour in 2 tablespoons of the olive oil; tilt the pan to coat evenly. Place the oiled pan back in the oven to heat for 2 more minutes. (This step ensures a crispy crust on the falafel.)

Using a fork, carefully transfer the falafel patties to the hot baking sheet and gently flatten them with your fingers to make 2-inch patties. Bake for 5 minutes; flip the patties and bake for 5 to 6 more minutes, until they start to turn golden.

While the patties cook, squeeze about 1 tablespoon of lemon juice into a medium bowl. Add the yogurt, remaining 1 tablespoon tahini, and remaining 1 teaspoon olive oil; whisk together.

To assemble the wraps, into the center of each flatbread place a spoonful of the tahini sauce, ¼ cup of the parsley, 3 falafel patties, tomato slices, and a squeeze of juice from the remaining lemon half. Fold up the bottom part of the wrap, then fold over each side and serve.

Healthy Kitchen Hack: Mediterranean dishes often feature cupfuls of fresh herbs versus meager tablespoons. Using an abundance of fresh herbs is a terrific way to add extra nutrients, color, and fresh flavor to any dish (not to mention a great way to use them up before they go bad). Match the amount of lettuce or spinach in your salad with equal cups of mint or basil leaves. Toss at least a cup of chopped cilantro or parsley (leaves and stems!) into soups, stews, or bean dishes toward the end of their cooking time. Blend your favorite green herb into yogurt dips for a vibrant color or even into smoothies. We usually pass on the green smoothies, but we can't resist the combo of fresh cilantro blended with frozen mango, orange juice, and vanilla yogurt.

Per Serving: Calories: 330; Total Fat: 13g; Saturated Fat: 2g; Cholesterol: 3mg; Sodium: 734mg; Total Carbohydrates: 44g; Fiber: 11g; Protein: 17g

Spanakopita Grilled Cheese Panini

| Nut-Free, Egg-Free, Vegetarian | Serves 4 | Prep time: 10 minutes | Cook time: 25 minutes |

1 tablespoon extra-virgin olive oil

½ cup chopped green onions

2 garlic cloves, minced

1 teaspoon dried oregano

¼ teaspoon black pepper

4 cups frozen chopped spinach (see Healthy Kitchen Hack below)

1 medium lemon, cut in half

½ cup crumbled feta cheese (2 ounces)

1 whole-grain Italian loaf, cut into 4 equal lengths

½ cup shredded part-skim mozzarella cheese (2 ounces)

Serena's children do not eat spinach. Ever. Not cooked or raw. They do not eat it (Sam-I-Am!). But during the testing of this recipe, every single one of Serena's four children asked for the second half of their panini (as Serena had only served them half to begin with—expecting the anti-spinach gene to prevail). So, serve up these sandwiches—inspired by spanakopita, the Greek spinach, onion, and cheese savory pie—and expect cheers for the two types of cheese *and* the spinach.

In a large skillet, heat the olive oil over medium-high heat. Add the green onions and cook, stirring occasionally, until softened, about 3 minutes. Add the garlic, oregano, and black pepper and cook, stirring frequently, for 30 seconds. Add the spinach and 3 tablespoons water and cook, stirring occasionally to break up any frozen chunks, until the liquid is mostly dissolved, 7 to 8 minutes. Turn off the heat and squeeze 1 tablespoon of lemon juice into the skillet. (Save any remaining lemon for another use.) Add the feta cheese and gently mix all the ingredients together.

Coat a panini maker, grill pan, or large skillet with cooking spray and heat over medium-high heat.

Cut open each section of bread horizontally, but don't cut all the way through. Fill each bread section with the spinach mixture, then top with the mozzarella cheese. Close the sandwiches and place two on the panini press, pan, or skillet. If using a panini press, close and grill until the crust is golden and the cheese has melted, 3 to 5 minutes. For a pan or skillet, place another skillet or a heavy object on top and grill for about 3 minutes. Flip and grill for another 2 to 3 minutes. Repeat with the other two sandwiches.

Healthy Kitchen Hack: While a bag of fresh spinach can easily be substituted for frozen in this recipe, we've discovered that frozen spinach "ain't what it used to be"—meaning the cumbersome solid ice block sold in 10-ounce boxes. Flash-freezing technology has improved, so today's chopped spinach is frozen as individual leaves, which makes it easy to measure out for recipes and allows it to thaw faster, too. It's also being sold in bags, making it that much easier to put the remaining frozen spinach back in the freezer for another use.

Per Serving: Calories: 345; Total Fat: 10g; Saturated Fat: 4g; Cholesterol: 22mg; Sodium: 644mg; Total Carbohydrates: 44g; Fiber: 11g; Protein: 19g

Grilled Veggie Gyros with Tzatziki Sauce

Nut-Free, Egg-Free, Vegetarian	**Serves 4**	Prep time: 20 minutes	Cook time: 10 minutes

1 small globe eggplant

1 small zucchini (3 to 4 ounces)

1 red onion

2 tablespoons extra-virgin olive oil

3 teaspoons dried oregano, divided

½ teaspoon kosher or sea salt, divided

¼ teaspoon black pepper

¼ teaspoon smoked paprika

1 cucumber

¾ cup plain 2% Greek yogurt (6 ounces)

½ cup chopped fresh dill

1 garlic clove, minced

½ cup crumbled goat cheese (2 ounces)

2 (6-inch) whole-wheat pita breads, toasted and cut into halves

1 roasted red pepper (from a 12-ounce jar or homemade—see page 44) drained and sliced

In the Greek gyro shops Serena visited on her honeymoon, the meat was very thinly sliced off a large spit of rotating meat. In our vegetarian version of the gyro, we replicate those strips with flavorful slices of roasted vegetables. We use herb goat cheese as a nod toward the herb-roasted goat meat often used in gyros and then finish the wraps off with a drizzle of the traditional tzatziki, a creamy yogurt-and-cucumber sauce.

Place one oven rack 3 to 4 inches below the broiler. Preheat the broiler to high for at least 5 minutes. Coat a large rimmed baking sheet with cooking spray.

Place the eggplant and zucchini on a cutting board and slice off the stem ends. Slice four ¼-inch-thick slices lengthwise from the middle of each vegetable. Slice the onion in half from root end to stem end, then slice one half of the onion into ¾-inch wedges, keeping the stem end intact so each wedge doesn't separate. (Save the remaining parts of the vegetables for another use—see our Healthy Kitchen Hack opposite for lots of ideas!)

In a large bowl, mix the olive oil, 2 teaspoons of the oregano, ¼ teaspoon of the salt, the black pepper, and the smoked paprika. Add the onion and toss to coat. Using a slotted spoon (or your hands) place the onion on the baking sheet, leaving most of the oil mixture in the bowl. Add zucchini and eggplant slices to the bowl and toss to coat. Place on the baking sheet, arranging them so there is room for the heat to circulate between the pieces. Broil for 3 to 4 minutes, until the vegetables begin to brown. Remove from the oven and turn over the vegetables. Place back under the broiler, repositioning the pan if necessary so all the vegetables cook evenly. Broil for another 3 to 4 minutes, until the vegetables begin to brown on the other side.

While the vegetables cook, cut the cucumber in half crosswise. Shred one half with a box grater (or finely chop with a knife). Add to a small bowl with the yogurt, dill, garlic, and the remaining salt and whisk together. Slice the remaining half of the cucumber into ¼-inch-thick slices and set aside.

Into a small bowl, put the goat cheese and the remaining 1 teaspoon oregano and mix together.

To assemble the gyros, into each pita, layer a few slices of cucumber, the roasted vegetables, and slices of roasted red pepper. Drizzle with the tzatziki sauce and sprinkle with the goat cheese.

Healthy Kitchen Hack: The great thing about having leftover veggies from the recipes in this book is that many of them will slide seamlessly right into another recipe. For example, the leftover zucchini, eggplant, and onion (and even the goat cheese) here will make one delicious Zucchini–Goat Cheese Pizza on page 136. And leftover veggies like zucchini, eggplant, kale, greens, onions, broccoli, cauliflower, and so on can always be used to make simple vegetable soups. Cook everything together in broth, then (carefully) puree the hot soup. Add a drizzle of olive oil, some leftover herbs, and a sprinkle of cheese. You can also use leftover veggies in stews, scrambled eggs, and grilled cheese sandwiches.

Per Serving: Calories: 280; Total Fat: 12g; Saturated Fat: 4g; Cholesterol: 11mg; Sodium: 455mg; Total Carbohydrates: 34g; Fiber: 5g; Protein: 13g

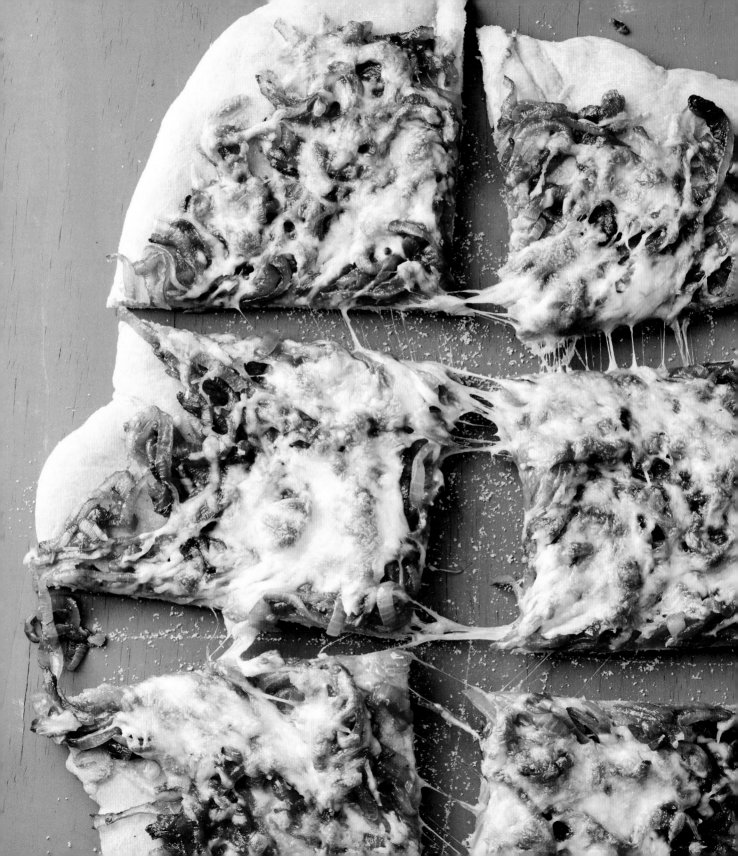

pizza

No-Rise Pizza Dough

Dairy-Free, Nut-Free, Egg-Free, Vegetarian   Serves 6   Prep time: 20 minutes

1½ cups all-purpose flour, plus more for kneading

1½ cups white whole-wheat flour

1 tablespoon baking powder

½ teaspoon kosher or sea salt

10 to 12 ounces beer

You can have pizza from scratch—including the dough—in less time than it takes to call for takeout. In this quickie pizza dough recipe, beer is the magical ingredient that replaces the yeast, which eliminates the hours you'd usually need for rising yet maintains the yeasty aromas of traditional pizza dough. It's our go-to crust for several recipes in this book, including Quick-Caramelized Onion Pizza (page 141) and Zucchini-Goat Cheese Pizza (page 136).

Into a large bowl, measure the flours, baking powder, and salt. Using a fork, mix together. Pour in a few ounces of beer at a time, mixing with a wooden spoon or rubber scraper in between each pour. Continue until a soft, but not sticky, dough ball forms (you will probably not use all of the beer).

Dust your countertop with all-purpose flour and add the dough. Knead for 1 to 2 minutes, until smooth, adding a few more teaspoons of flour if needed.

Roll the dough out into your preferred shape and let it rest for 10 minutes. Use in your favorite pizza recipe calling for 1 pound of dough. The dough can also be shaped into six equal pieces for individual pizzas. If not using immediately, place in a zip-top freezer bag or freezer-safe container and freeze for up to 6 months. To defrost, remove from the freezer and (leaving it in the bag or container) keep on the countertop for 2 to 3 hours, until completely thawed.

Healthy Kitchen Hack: White whole-wheat flour has a milder taste than traditional (darker-colored) whole-wheat flour but has all the nutritional benefits of a whole grain. When substituting any whole-wheat flour for all-purpose flour, try equal parts all-purpose flour and whole-wheat flour.

Per Serving: Calories: 242; Total Fat: 1g; Saturated Fat: 0g; Cholesterol: 0mg; Sodium: 165mg; Total Carbohydrates: 49g; Fiber: 4g; Protein: 8g

Socca Pizza with Shrimp and Leeks

Dairy-Free, Nut-Free, Gluten-Free, Egg-Free	Serves 4	Prep time: 10 minutes	Cook time: 30 minutes

¾ cup sliced leek (from ½ leek)

4 tablespoons extra-virgin olive oil, divided

1 cup chickpea (garbanzo bean) flour

½ teaspoon black pepper, divided

¼ teaspoon kosher salt

2 teaspoons chopped fresh rosemary or ¾ teaspoon dried

½ cup Easy Roasted Tomato Sauce (page 147)

8 ounces frozen medium shrimp, thawed, peeled, and tails removed

¼ cup chopped fresh basil leaves

Back in the summer of 1993 (before cell phones, email, and the Internet), Deanna backpacked across Europe with college girlfriends. Despite their frugal travel budget, she felt like she ate like a queen by sampling new foods and local dishes from street vendors. Socca—a simple chickpea flatbread from Nice, France, is one street food she'll never forget. Cooked on a gigantic skillet over a steel drum fire, it was cut into slices and served with lots of black pepper. Here, Deanna re-created the recipe to use as a gluten-free pizza crust, but one you'll need to eat with a fork and knife as it's a bit too delicate to pick up with your hands.

Preheat the oven to 450°F.

Put the leeks and 1 tablespoon of the olive oil into a 10-inch cast iron skillet. Stir a few times and place in the oven. Roast for 5 minutes, stirring once.

While the leeks cook, in a large bowl, put the chickpea flour, 2 tablespoons of the olive oil, the rosemary, ¼ teaspoon of the black pepper, and the salt. Whisk together and then slowly pour in ¾ cup warm water, mixing until a thin batter is formed. Set aside.

Remove the skillet from the oven and spoon the leeks into the batter. Set the hot skillet on the stovetop, keeping an oven mitt on the handle (to remind you it's hot!). Mix the leeks into the batter and pour the batter into the skillet. Spread the batter around so it reaches all sides of the skillet. Return the skillet to the oven and bake the socca for 10 minutes.

Remove the skillet and brush the top of the socca with the remaining 1 tablespoon olive oil. Spread the tomato sauce evenly over the top. (If you prefer a smoother tomato sauce, puree it first.) Return the skillet to the oven and bake the socca for 10 more minutes.

continued

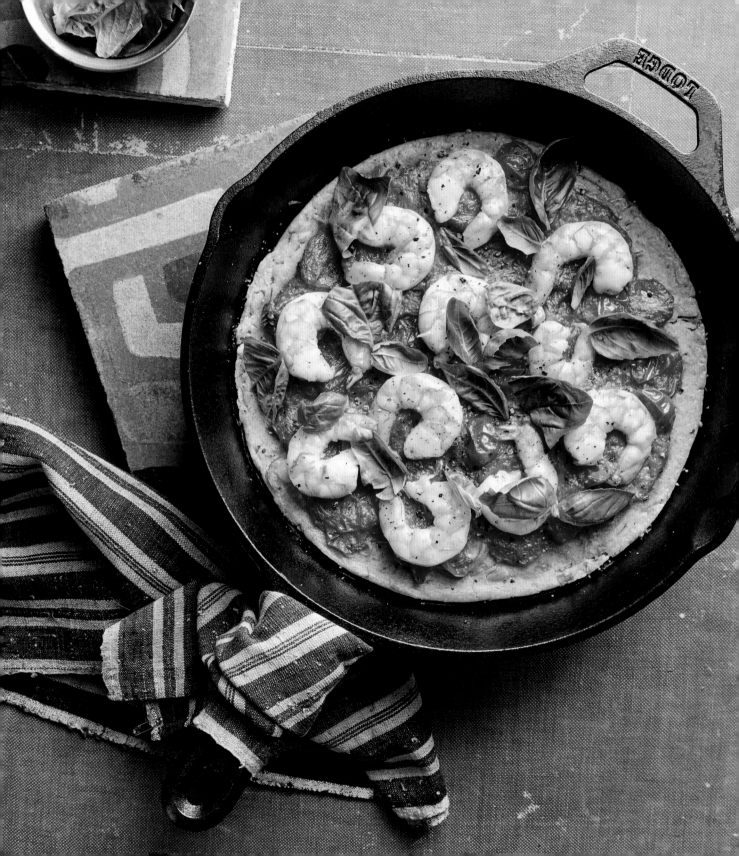

Socca Pizza with Shrimp and Leeks (continued)

Open the oven door, pull out the rack using oven mitts, and sprinkle the shrimp over top of the tomato sauce. Sprinkle with the remaining ¼ teaspoon black pepper. Bake for 5 more minutes, until the shrimp just turn pink and start to curl. Remove from the oven and sprinkle with the basil. Cool slightly before cutting and serving (keeping an oven mitt on the skillet handle, as it will remain hot to the touch for a bit).

Healthy Kitchen Hack: Use this socca crust as a base for your other favorite pizza toppings. Or instead of topping the socca, brush it with a few more teaspoons of olive oil and continue to cook according to the recipe instructions. Slice and serve as a gluten-free bread option at meals.

Per Serving: Calories: 279; Total Fat: 16g; Saturated Fat: 2g; Cholesterol: 91mg; Sodium: 210mg; Total Carbohydrates: 18g; Fiber: 3g; Protein: 17g

"My entire family thought this was absolutely delicious! When paired with a salad, it was a light dinner for four."

—Jessica from Silver Spring, MD

Mushroom-Sausage Stromboli

Nut-Free		Serves 6	Prep time: 20 minutes	Cook time: 20 minutes

1 pound refrigerated or thawed frozen pizza dough, at room temperature

2 cups white mushrooms (8 ounces)

6 ounces 70% lean ground pork

1 garlic clove, minced

3 teaspoons fresh thyme leaves or 1 teaspoon dried, divided

¾ cup shredded mozzarella cheese (about 3 ounces)

1 large egg

1 (24-ounce) jar low-sodium tomato sauce

Mushrooms add rich, savory flavors to this stromboli and mix in seamlessly with the ground pork here so you can use less meat. It's Serena's favorite dinner to bring to new parents or a friend in need. Simply wrap it up in the parchment paper after baking and add a bag of green salad with some pieces of fresh fruit for a complete meal ready to deliver (but so much better than pizza delivery!).

Preheat the oven to 425°F. Line a large rimmed baking sheet with parchment paper.

Using your hands, stretch and press the dough into a 12 by 8-inch rectangle on the counter, then transfer it to the prepared baking sheet.

Using a food processor, pulse the mushrooms until they resemble the texture of ground meat—but not so much that they turn into a puree. (Or finely chop the mushrooms with a knife.)

In a large skillet over medium-high heat, cook the mushrooms, pork, garlic, and 1½ teaspoons of the fresh thyme (or ½ teaspoon dried), stirring occasionally until no pink remains in the pork and most of the liquid released by the mushrooms evaporates, 6 to 8 minutes. Using a slotted spoon, remove the mushroom-pork mixture to a paper towel–lined plate to drain.

The pizza dough will have shrunk, so press it again into a 12 by 8-inch rectangle. Spoon the mushroom-mixture down the center of the dough lengthwise, leaving a 1½-inch border at the ends (the filling should be in a line about 9 inches long). Sprinkle the cheese on top of the filling. Fold one-third of the dough over the filling and then fold the other third over so it overlaps the first fold of the dough. Pinch to seal all the edges.

Into a small bowl, crack the egg and add 2 teaspoons water. Whisk together and then brush the egg wash over the entire stromboli. Sprinkle with the remaining 1½ teaspoons fresh thyme (or ½ teaspoon dried).

continued

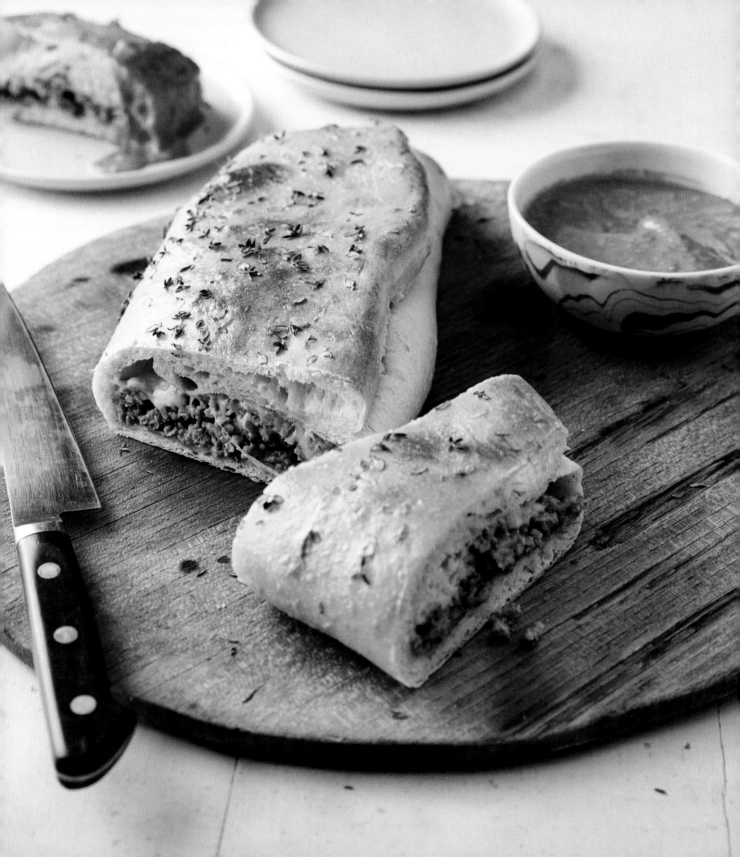

Mushroom-Sausage Stromboli (continued)

Bake for 20 minutes or until the stromboli turns golden.

Cut into 6 slices and serve hot or at room temperature with the pasta sauce for dipping.

Healthy Kitchen Hack: Use a "blend" of mushrooms and ground meat whenever you want to extend ground meat to make it more budget friendly and nutrient rich. Add chopped mushrooms to any recipe calling for ground meat, such as meatballs, tacos, chili, or sausage breakfast casseroles. Raw or cooked (and cooled) mushrooms can be added in almost any ratio: use 8 ounces of mushrooms and the same amount of meat, or use more meat than mushrooms as we did here. This mushroom hack helps retain juiciness, which is especially important when cooking lower-fat varieties of ground beef, pork, lamb, chicken, and turkey.

Per Serving: Calories: 273; Total Fat: 9g; Saturated Fat: 4g; Cholesterol: 30mg; Sodium: 574mg; Total Carbohydrates: 35g; Fiber: 3g; Protein: 13g

Green Olive Pita Pizzas

Nut-Free, Egg-Free, Vegetarian	Serves 4	Prep time: 5 minutes	Cook time: 5 minutes

4 (7- to 8-inch) whole-wheat pita breads

2 teaspoons extra-virgin olive oil

½ cup jarred low-sodium tomato pasta sauce or Easy Roasted Tomato Sauce (page 147)

1 large fresh mozzarella ball (about 4 ounces total), thinly sliced

1 (6-ounce) can or jar whole green olives (about 1¼ cups), rinsed and sliced

1 tablespoon grated Parmesan or Pecorino Romano cheese

¼ teaspoon dried oregano leaves

For the days when Deanna doesn't even have time for No-Rise Pizza Dough (page 128), she uses pita bread to make individual pizzas in minutes. She's always preferred the buttery, milder-flavored green olives to the black ones, and was giddy to find green olive–topped pizza at a small Israeli pizza joint during her trip. Seek out canned green olives at your store so you can taste their true smooth flavor, as they aren't soaked in an acidic brine as the jarred variety are.

Preheat the broiler to high. Coat a large rimmed baking sheet with cooking spray. Place the pita breads on the baking sheet and brush with the olive oil. Spoon the tomato sauce onto each pita and spread with the back of the spoon. Top with the mozzarella and sliced olives. Sprinkle with the Parmesan and oregano.

Broil for 2 to 2½ minutes, until the cheese is melted and the edges of the pita start to crisp. Remove from the oven and cut each pita into 6 wedges before serving.

Healthy Kitchen Hack: Canned or jarred, olives are preserved with a decent amount of salt. To remove some of the sodium, we drain them in a strainer and then rinse them under running water. But before draining, look to see if your recipe calls for using some of the liquid so you can save it before it goes down the drain.

Per Serving: Calories: 319; Total Fat: 13g; Saturated Fat: 4g; Cholesterol: 11mg; Sodium: 826mg; Total Carbohydrates: 40g; Fiber: 6g; Protein: 13g

Zucchini–Goat Cheese Pizza

Nut-Free, Egg-Free, Vegetarian	Serves 6	Prep time:10 minutes	Cook time: 20 minutes

1 pound refrigerated (or thawed frozen) pizza dough or No-Rise Pizza Dough (page 128), at room temperature

1 tablespoon extra-virgin olive oil

2 small or 1 medium zucchini, (7 to 8 ounces total) thinly sliced into half circles

½ small red onion, thinly sliced

2 garlic cloves, minced

⅛ teaspoon crushed red pepper (optional)

1 medium lemon, cut in half

¼ teaspoon black pepper

1 large fresh mozzarella balls (about 4 ounces total), chopped

4 ounces goat cheese, crumbled

3 tablespoons fresh basil leaves, torn

Zucchini is abundant throughout Mediterranean cuisine—it's served grilled, baked, stuffed, and sautéed, and can be paired with just about any savory ingredient. Deanna was experimenting with some different pizza toppings one day and came up with this heavenly combo—zucchini with red onions, goat cheese, and fresh mozzarella. Along with zucchini noodles (pages 164 and 250), she now makes this zucchini dish all summer long.

Preheat the oven to 500°F. Coat a large rimmed baking sheet with cooking spray.

On a lightly floured surface, form the pizza dough into a 12-inch circle, using a rolling pin or stretching it with your hands. Place the dough on the prepared baking sheet and set aside.

In a large skillet over medium-high heat, heat the olive oil. Add the zucchini and onion and cook, stirring frequently, until the vegetables start to soften, 5 minutes. Add the garlic and crushed red pepper (if using). Cook, stirring constantly, for 30 seconds. Squeeze 1 tablespoon of lemon juice into the skillet. (Save any remaining lemon for another use.) Add the black pepper and stir. Remove from the heat.

Spread the topping evenly on the pizza dough, leaving a ½-inch border. Top with the mozzarella and goat cheese. Bake for 10 to 12 minutes, until the cheese is melted and the crust starts to brown around the edges.

Remove from the oven and slide onto a wooden cutting board. Top with the torn basil and then cut into 6 pieces.

Healthy Kitchen Hack: When you find yourself with extra zucchini, you can double this topping and turn it into a side dish. Cook the zucchini, onion, and garlic according to the instructions. Mix in the lemon juice, season with salt and pepper, and serve without the cheese. Or mix all the ingredients together and toss with your favorite cooked pasta. It is also yummy as a topping for cooked chicken or fish.

Per Serving: Calories: 365; Total Fat: 12g; Saturated Fat: 5g; Cholesterol: 40mg; Sodium: 765mg; Total Carbohydrates: 46g; Protein: 17g

Garlic and Mushroom Lovers' Flatbread Pizza

| Nut-Free, Vegetarian | Serves 4 | Prep time: 15 minutes | Cook time: 25 minutes |

3 tablespoons yellow cornmeal

¾ cup all-purpose flour

¾ cup white whole-wheat flour

1 tablespoon dried oregano

½ teaspoon baking powder

¾ teaspoon kosher or sea salt, divided

1 cup plus 2 tablespoons reduced-fat (2%) milk

2 large eggs

1 tablespoon extra-virgin olive oil

3 cups sliced white mushrooms

5 garlic cloves, thinly sliced

1 tablespoon white wine vinegar or red wine vinegar

¾ cup grated Parmesan or Pecorino Romano cheese (about 4 ounces)

Our favorite way to make pizza on the fly is to *pour* the dough into a pan. The crust is a bit of a mash-up of Serena's two pizza loves: soft Chicago-style deep-dish and a super-thin St. Louis style. Add the classic Mediterranean combo of meaty mushrooms with aromatic garlic and it's a perfect pizza pie or flatbread!

Place an oven rack about 4 inches below the broiler. Preheat the oven to 400°F. Coat a large rimmed baking sheet with cooking spray. Sprinkle the baking sheet with the cornmeal; turn and tap the baking sheet to spread the cornmeal evenly.

Into a large bowl, measure the flours, oregano, baking powder, and ½ teaspoon of the salt and mix together. In a small bowl, whisk together the milk and eggs. Add to the flour mixture and mix until well combined.

Pour the batter onto the prepared baking sheet and tilt the baking sheet to spread the batter evenly.

Bake for 10 to 12 minutes, until the crust appears dry in the center. Remove from the oven and turn the broiler on high.

While the crust cooks, in a large skillet over medium heat, heat the olive oil. Add the mushrooms and garlic and cook, stirring frequently, until the mushrooms start to shrink, 5 to 7 minutes. Add the vinegar and the remaining ¼ teaspoon salt; stir and cook until most of the liquid evaporates, about 3 more minutes.

Evenly spread the mushroom mixture over the baked pizza crust. Sprinkle with the Parmesan cheese.

Place the pizza on the upper oven rack under the broiler. Broil, rotating the pan halfway through (and watching carefully to prevent burning), for 2 to 3 minutes, until the cheese is melted and golden.

Healthy Kitchen Hack: Turn this recipe into one of the most popular appetizers on our blog, TeaspoonOfSpice.com. To make our Bacon Onion Tart, use this crust recipe and top with the onions from our Quick-Caramelized Onion Pizza (page 141). Add some chopped bacon, grated cheese, and chopped chives. To serve, cut into small squares.

Per Serving: Calories: 386; Total Fat: 14g; Saturated Fat: 5g; Cholesterol: 115mg; Sodium: 775mg; Total Carbohydrates: 49g; Fiber: 5g; Protein: 19g

"I thought the toppings were fantastic; they're a great blend of flavors with the garlic, mushrooms, and red wine vinegar. I've made it several times and once I added spinach when sautéing the mushrooms, which turned out well, too!"

—Rachel from St. Paul, MN

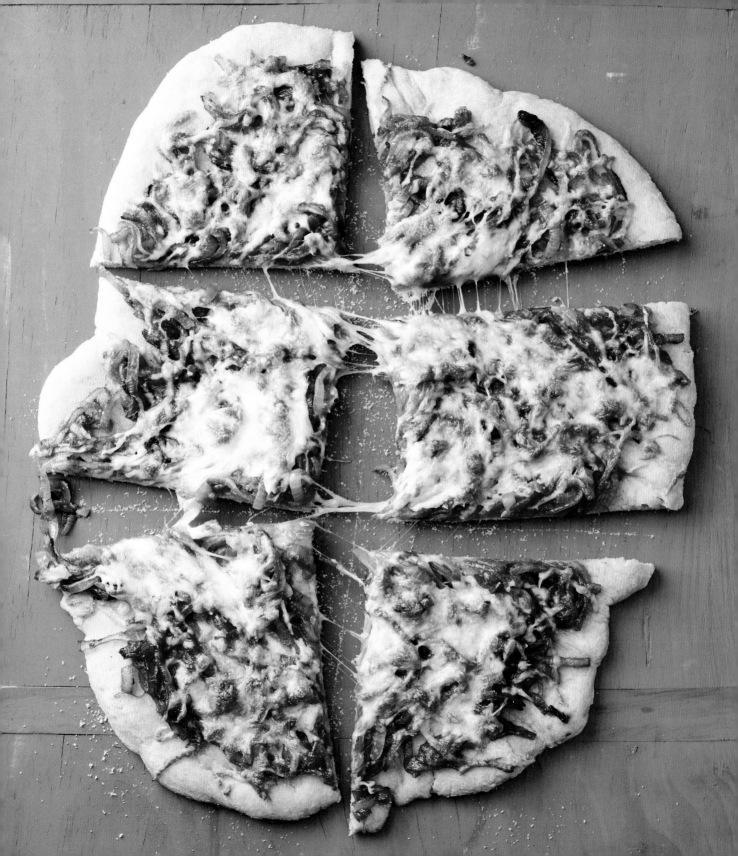

Quick-Caramelized Onion Pizza

Nut-Free, Egg-Free, Vegetarian	Serves 6	Prep time: 10 minutes	Cook time: 30 minutes

1 tablespoon cornmeal

3 medium yellow onions (about 1 pound)

2 tablespoons plus 2 teaspoons extra-virgin olive oil, divided

¼ teaspoon kosher or sea salt

¼ teaspoon black pepper

1 pound refrigerated or thawed frozen pizza dough or No-Rise Pizza Dough (page 128), at room temperature

1 cup shredded part-skim mozzarella cheese (4 ounces)

If you've never eaten caramelized onions straight out of the pan (or off of a pizza,) you're missing out. This recipe has not one but *two* ways to make caramelized onions—that's how badly we want you to make this savory-sweet way to add giant flavor to everything from sandwiches and pasta to dips and, of course, pizza. Or, as we said, you could just eat them with a spoon.

Preheat the oven to 450°F. Coat a large rimmed baking sheet with cooking spray and sprinkle with the cornmeal.

Slice each onion in half from the bulb end to the root end. Once halved, it will be easier to peel off the papery skins. Peel and then slice into very thin half-moons (about ⅛ inch thick).

Heat a large skillet over medium heat, then pour in 2 tablespoons of the olive oil. Add the onions to the pan. Cook for 10 minutes, stirring occasionally to break apart the onion slices. Check the color after 10 minutes of cooking time; if they are beginning to brown you can remove them from the stove, but they will develop a richer flavor if they are cooked an additional 10 to 15 minutes longer, stirring occasionally. When the onions are brown and caramelized with a few very dark (almost burnt) onions, add 2 tablespoons water and the salt and black pepper. Stir and scrape up the dark bits on the bottom of the skillet. Cook until the liquid evaporates, about 2 minutes.

While the onions cook, press the dough into an oval or rectangle about ½ inch thick on the prepared baking sheet. Drizzle the remaining 2 teaspoons oil over the dough and spread with your fingers. Bake for 5 minutes and then remove from the oven.

Scatter the onions onto the partially baked dough. Top with the cheese. Bake for 8 to 10 minutes until the crust is golden.

continued

Quick-Caramelized Onion Pizza (continued)

Healthy Kitchen Hack: Caramelized onions are one of our favorite ways to add a contrast of bold flavors (and more veggies!) to any dish. Make a batch on the stovetop or use your slow cooker for a totally hands-off approach. Add 1½ to 2 pounds thinly sliced onions to a cooking spray–coated slow cooker. Sprinkle with 2 tablespoons extra-virgin olive oil and ½ teaspoon kosher salt. Cover and cook on high for 4 hours or on low for 6 to 8 hours. No stirring is required!

Per Serving: Calories: 308; Total Fat: 10g; Saturated Fat: 3g; Cholesterol: 9mg; Sodium: 532mg; Total Carbohydrates: 45g; Fiber: 3g; Protein: 8g

Fig-Prosciutto Focaccia

Nut-Free, Egg-Free		Serves 8	Prep time: 10 minutes	Cook time: 20 minutes

4 tablespoons extra-virgin olive oil, divided

1 pound refrigerated or thawed frozen pizza dough, at room temperature

3 garlic cloves, minced

1 tablespoon finely chopped fresh rosemary leaves

10 dried figs, sliced into circles

2 large fresh mozzarella balls (about 8 ounces total), cut into ¼-inch slices

1 ounce prosciutto, sliced into 1-inch pieces

¼ teaspoon black pepper

Sweet, plump figs paired with salty, cured meats is a match made in pizza heaven. The Mediterranean region (and California in the US) has the perfect climate for growing many varieties. When fresh figs are in season (usually a few weeks in late summer), treat yourself! Then use them here—if you haven't already eaten them all out of hand.

Preheat the oven to 450°F. Brush a large rimmed baking sheet with 1 tablespoon of the olive oil.

On a work surface, stretch the dough with your hands or use a rolling pin to shape it into a 16×12-inch rectangle. Then arrange the dough on the prepared baking sheet, pushing the dough into all the corners. Dimple the dough by pressing down using your knuckles or fingertips to leave deep indentations. Bake for 8 minutes.

While the crust cooks, heat a small skillet over medium-low heat. Pour in the remaining 3 tablespoons olive oil and add the garlic and rosemary. Cook, stirring frequently, for 3 minutes. Remove from the stove.

Remove the focaccia crust from the oven, drizzle with the infused oil, and brush to evenly coat. Add the sliced figs on top, pressing them slightly into the dough. Top with the mozzarella and prosciutto. Sprinkle with the black pepper. Bake for 8 to 10 minutes, until the edges just start to crisp and the cheese is melted. Remove from the oven and cut into 8 pieces.

Healthy Kitchen Hack: Instead of using tomato sauce, make a fig "pizza" sauce! Add ¾ cup chopped dried figs to a saucepan with 1½ cups water. Bring to a boil and then reduce the heat to medium-low. Simmer until the liquid reduces by half, about 15 minutes. Puree in a blender with 1 teaspoon honey and ¼ teaspoon kosher or sea salt. Spread half onto precooked pizza dough before adding any toppings. Refrigerate the remaining sauce for up to a week.

Per Serving: Calories: 305; Total Fat: 15g; Saturated Fat: 5g; Cholesterol: 11mg; Sodium: 481mg; Total Carbohydrates: 32g; Fiber: 1g; Protein: 11g

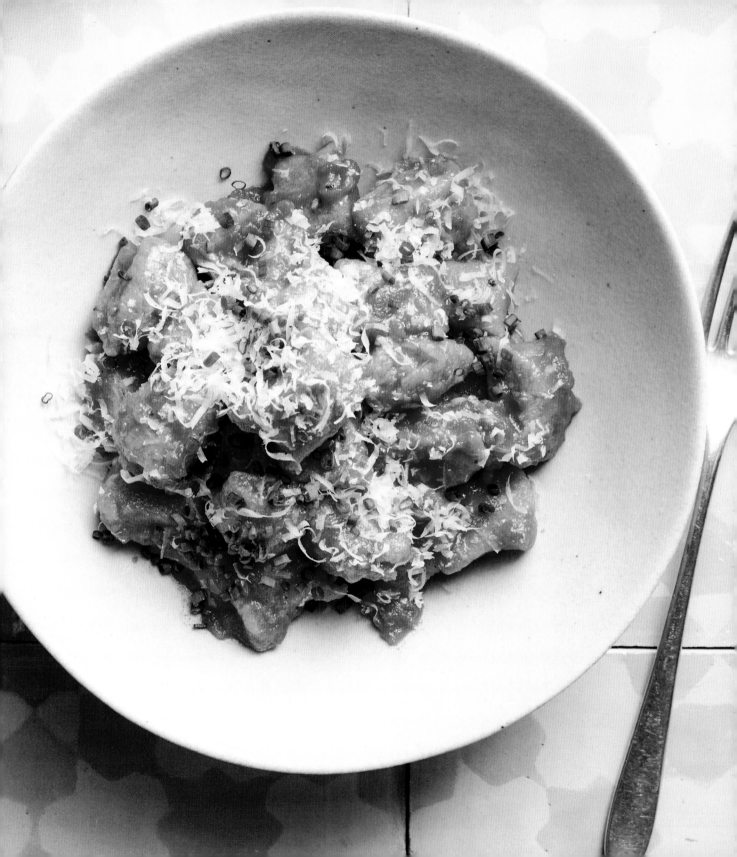

pasta

Oven-Baked Spinach-Feta Gnocchi

| Nut-Free, Egg-Free, Vegetarian | Serves 4 | Prep time: 5 minutes | Cook time: 20 minutes |

1 pound frozen gnocchi

2½ cups frozen chopped spinach

¾ cup crumbled feta cheese (3 ounces)

3 tablespoons extra-virgin olive oil

¼ cup chopped green onions

3 garlic cloves, minced

¼ teaspoon ground nutmeg

¼ teaspoon kosher or sea salt

¼ teaspoon black pepper

1½ tablespoons grated Parmesan or Pecorino Romano cheese

For spinach dip fans, this is a must-make meal. From freezer to oven, this pasta dinner couldn't be easier to whip up. Deanna recently discovered that frozen gnocchi cooks up beautifully in the oven—no pot of boiling water needed!

Preheat the oven to 450°F.

Onto a 9×11- or 9×13-inch metal baking pan, put the frozen gnocchi, frozen spinach, feta, olive oil, green onions, garlic, nutmeg, salt, and black pepper. Gently mix all the ingredients together with your hands.

Bake for 15 minutes, stirring once halfway through the cooking time. Carefully pull out the oven rack and add 1 cup water to the pan. Stir and then sprinkle with the Parmesan cheese. Bake for 5 more minutes, until a thick sauce forms. Remove from the oven and stir a few times before serving. (The sauce will continue to thicken as it sits.)

Healthy Kitchen Hack: For our artichoke dip fans, adding a can of artichokes to this recipe takes this dinner to new flavor heights along with adding 5 grams of fiber and even more veggies per serving. Drain one (14-ounce) can of artichoke hearts, chop, and mix into the gnocchi with the other ingredients before putting the pan in the oven.

Per Serving: Calories: 438; Total Fat: 19g; Saturated Fat: 6g; Cholesterol: 34mg; Sodium: 552mg; Total Carbohydrates: 55g; Fiber: 4g; Protein: 16g

Easy Roasted Tomato Sauce

Dairy-Free, Nut-Free, Gluten-Free, Egg-Free, Vegan	Serves 4	Prep time: 10 minutes	Cook time: 20 minutes

2 large tomatoes or 1 quart grape tomatoes, chopped (about 3 cups)

2 tablespoons chopped fresh thyme, rosemary, or oregano, or 2 teaspoons dried

1½ tablespoons extra-virgin olive oil

2 garlic cloves, minced

1 teaspoon smoked paprika or ¼ teaspoon crushed red pepper

¼ teaspoon kosher or sea salt

¼ teaspoon black pepper

"The recipe is super clear to follow, simple to make, and incredibly flavorful, especially with fresh basil. And I love the idea of turning it into a soup!"

—Jessica from Silver Spring, MD

Of all the recipes in the cookbook, this is the one that Deanna has been making the longest and still cooks up almost weekly. It's a great way to use up the bumper tomato crop in the summer or those older tomatoes during the rest of the year. In the off season, Deanna uses grape tomatoes, which work well in this application because they are less watery. Bonus nutrition tip: Cooking tomatoes in fat (here olive oil) enhances our bodies' ability to absorb lycopene, the antioxidant that gives tomatoes their red color and is linked to lowering the risk of prostate cancer.

Preheat the oven to 425°F.

Put all the ingredients onto a 9×13-inch baking pan. Mix well and place in the oven. Roast the sauce, stirring a few times, for 18 to 20 minutes until the tomatoes soften and start to caramelize. For a smooth sauce, transfer to a blender and blend to the consistency you prefer. Use as a pasta or pizza sauce as we do with our Crispy Ravioli (page 155) or Socca Pizza with Shrimp and Leeks (page 129).

Healthy Kitchen Hack: For a zesty and unique pasta or pizza sauce, puree this tomato sauce with our Roasted Red Peppers (page 44) in a blender. Or for a quick vegan soup, mix this tomato pepper sauce with 1 cup low-sodium vegetable broth. Warm it up in a saucepan over medium heat.

Per Serving: Calories: 65; Total Fat: 6g; Saturated Fat: 1g; Cholesterol: 0mg; Sodium: 125mg; Total Carbohydrates: 4g; Fiber: 1g; Protein: 1g

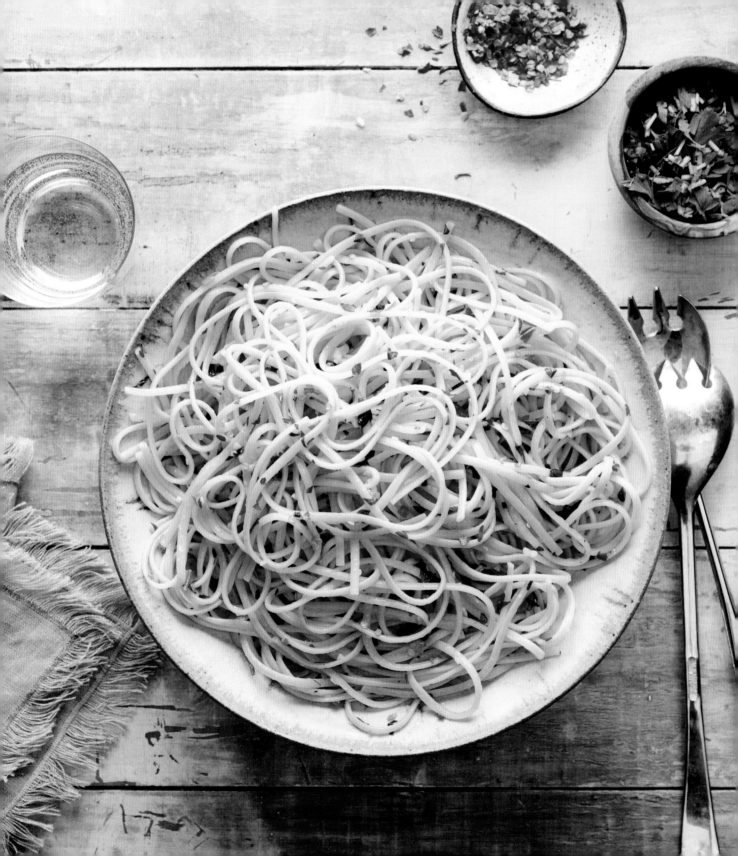

Spicy Linguine with Garlic and Oil (Aglio e Olio)

| Nut-Free, Egg-Free, Vegetarian | **Serves 6** | Prep time: 5 minutes | Cook time: 20 minutes |

1¾ teaspoons kosher or sea salt, divided

1 (16-ounce) package linguine or spaghetti

¼ cup extra-virgin olive oil

5 garlic cloves, minced

½ teaspoon crushed red pepper

½ cup chopped fresh parsley

¼ cup grated Parmesan or Pecorino Romano cheese

¼ teaspoon black pepper

Despite the short ingredient list, this classic and simple pasta dish packs a wallop of flavor from the garlic, crushed red pepper, parsley, and Parmesan. Whenever she makes pasta, Deanna usually does a mix of half regular and half whole-wheat noodles for some added nutrients and a bit of nutty flavor. At times, she'll also add cooked shrimp or salmon to this recipe for more protein and as a way to eat more seafood during the week.

Place a large stockpot filled with water on the stove and cover. Bring to a boil and add 1½ teaspoons of the salt. Cook the pasta according to the package instructions. Drain the pasta, reserving about ½ cup of the pasta water. Return the drained pasta with a few tablespoons of the pasta water back to the stockpot.

In a large skillet over medium heat, heat the olive oil. Add the garlic and crushed red pepper; cook, stirring frequently so as not to let the garlic burn, for 2 minutes. Add ¼ cup of the pasta water to the skillet; cook, stirring occasionally, to make a loose sauce, 2 minutes.

Add the cooked pasta to the skillet and mix together with tongs. Heat for 1 more minute.

Remove from the stove and add the parsley, cheese, remaining ¼ teaspoon salt, and the black pepper. Mix together one last time with tongs and serve.

Healthy Kitchen Hack: While your pasta-cooking water doesn't have to (and shouldn't!) taste like the ocean as you may have heard, it is essential to add salt to the water or your cooked pasta will taste completely bland. The good news is that the majority of the salt is not absorbed into the cooked pasta, so your recipe's sodium levels won't be sky high. We found that 1½ teaspoons kosher or sea salt is the perfect amount to add to the pot of boiling water for one pound of pasta, which results in an addition of only about ⅛ teaspoon sodium to the entire recipe.

Per Serving: Calories: 386; Total Fat: 12g; Saturated Fat: 2g; Cholesterol: 4mg; Sodium: 616mg; Total Carbohydrates: 59g; Fiber: 3g; Protein: 11g

Pink Pasta Alfredo

Nut-Free, Egg-Free, Vegetarian	Serves 8	Prep time: 15 minutes	Cook time: 30 minutes

1 pound beets, peeled and cut into ¾-inch cubes, or 1 (15-ounce) can cooked beets, drained

2½ tablespoons extra-virgin olive oil, divided

2 teaspoons kosher or sea salt, divided

1 (16-ounce) package farfalle (bow-tie) or other medium or large pasta shape

1½ cups reduced-fat (2%) milk

½ teaspoon garlic powder

1½ tablespoons white whole-wheat flour

¾ cup grated Parmesan or Pecorino Romano cheese (about 2½ ounces), divided

½ teaspoon black pepper

Love noodles in a creamy sauce? This vibrant, hot-pink pasta may become your new favorite cheesy bowl of comfort food that also conveniently provides an extra serving of vegetables. Our trick is to make a three-ingredient white sauce and mix in pureed roasted beets. Or, if you prefer the color orange, try it with roasted carrots, butternut squash, or sweet potatoes. Winter root veggies are a big part of eating a seasonal Mediterranean Diet and this recipe presents them in a family-approved way!

Preheat the oven to 425°F. Spray a large rimmed baking sheet with cooking spray.

In a large bowl, toss the beets with 1 tablespoon of the olive oil and ¼ teaspoon of the salt. Spread the beets on the baking sheet and roast for 20 to 25 minutes, until a fork pierces the flesh easily. (If using canned beets, skip the cooking step.)

While the beets cook, place a large stockpot filled with water on the stove and cover. Bring to a boil and add 1½ teaspoons of the salt. Add the pasta and stir. Cook according to the package instructions. Drain the pasta, reserving ¾ cup of the pasta water. Return the drained pasta and 2 table-spoons of the pasta water to the stockpot.

While the pasta cooks, in a small microwave-safe bowl, warm the milk and garlic powder in the microwave for 1 minute. In a medium saucepan over medium heat, heat the remaining 1½ tablespoons olive oil. Whisk in the flour and cook for 1 minute, whisking constantly. In a slow, steady stream, whisk in the warm milk. Stir often until the mixture starts to bubble, then cook for 5 minutes more until thickened. If the pasta or beets aren't done, reduce the heat to low.

While the Alfredo sauce cooks, to a food processor, add the cooked beets and ¼ cup of the pasta water. Puree the beets until smooth. Measure out 1 cup of the beet puree. (Save the leftover puree in the refrigerator and stir it into tomato pasta sauce or chili.) Whisk the pureed beets into the Alfredo sauce until incorporated. Mix in ½ cup of the cheese.

continued

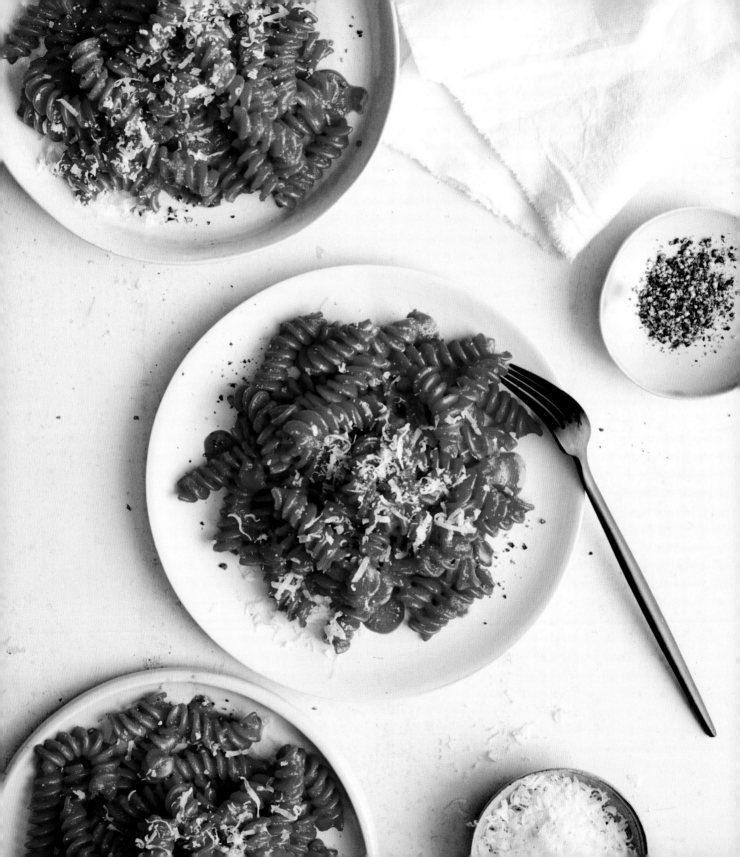

Place the cooked pasta in a large serving bowl. Add the beet-cheese sauce, the remaining ¼ teaspoon salt, and the black pepper. Toss gently to coat, adding more pasta water if needed to help the sauce coat the noodles. Sprinkle with the remaining ¼ cup cheese and serve.

Healthy Kitchen Hack: If you're like Serena, you may have wondered why pasta companies list the amount of water needed for cooking on the pasta box. It's because most people don't cook pasta in *enough* water; Serena didn't use enough water until Deanna and a few Italian chefs "schooled" her. If adequate water isn't used, adding the pasta will cool down the boiling water too much, which results in pasta that's mushy on the outside and undercooked on the inside. Additionally, the pasta cooking times listed on the package won't be accurate if sufficient water isn't used.

Per Serving: Calories: 338; Total Fat: 9g; Saturated Fat: 3g; Cholesterol: 10mg; Sodium: 370mg; Total Carbohydrates: 52g; Fiber: 4g; Protein: 13g

"This dish is so pretty—and almost shockingly pink. It's also a unique (and yummy!) way to get everyone to enjoy beets."

—Jo from Dickinson, ND

Penne with Almond Pesto and Eggplant

Egg-Free, Vegetarian	Serves 8	Prep time: 15 minutes	Cook time: 20 minutes

1½ teaspoons kosher or sea salt

1 (16-ounce) package penne pasta

¼ cup plus 2 tablespoons extra-virgin olive oil, divided

1 globe eggplant (about 1 pound), cut into ½-inch cubes

2 cups fresh basil leaves

¼ cup almonds

3 tablespoons grated Parmesan or Pecorino Romano cheese

2 garlic cloves

Dried penne pasta is a staple in Deanna's pantry because of the shape's versatility. Its "quill" form works well in soups, casseroles, mac 'n' cheese, and nearly any pasta dish, as sauces like pesto cling well to the hollow tubes.

Place a large stockpot filled with water on the stove and cover. Bring to a boil and add the salt. Add the penne and stir. Cook according to the package instructions. Drain the pasta, reserving a few tablespoons of the pasta water. Return the drained pasta and reserved pasta water to the stockpot.

While the pasta cooks, place a large skillet with 1 tablespoon of the olive oil over medium heat. Add half of the eggplant and cook until softened, stirring often, 8 to 10 minutes. Remove from the skillet and put in a large serving bowl. Add another 1 tablespoon of the olive oil to the pan and repeat the cooking process with the remaining eggplant.

In a food processor or blender, add the basil, almonds, cheese, and garlic. Process until roughly chopped. Scrape down the sides of the processor. Turn back on and slowly drizzle in the remaining ¼ cup olive oil. Process until smooth.

Add the cooked penne and pesto to the serving bowl with the eggplant. Toss well until all the pasta is coated with the pesto sauce.

Healthy Kitchen Hack: We love making pesto because it's a super-adaptable recipe that can be whipped up in seconds. Swap in whatever nuts (like almonds, pistachios, walnuts, peanuts, or pecans), grated aged cheese (use Parmesan, Pecorino Romano, or Asiago), and fresh herbs or delicate greens you have on hand (basil, mint, parsley, cilantro, spinach, or arugula). Use this formula with any combination of the ingredients suggested above: 2 cups greens, ¼ cup nuts, ¼ cup extra-virgin olive oil, 3 tablespoons grated aged cheese, and 2 garlic cloves. Add the ingredients to a blender or food processor and process until a thick and smooth sauce forms.

Per Serving: Calories: 355; Total Fat: 14g; Saturated Fat: 2g; Cholesterol: 1mg; Sodium: 67mg; Total Carbohydrates: 48g; Fiber: 5g; Protein: 10g

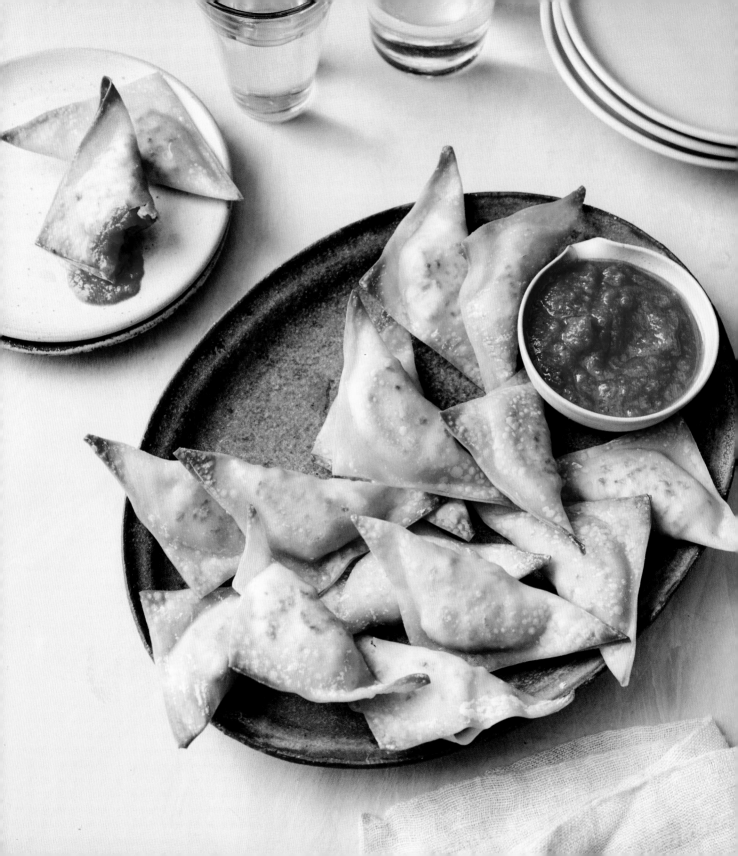

Crispy Ravioli with Tomato Dipping Sauce

Nut-Free, Egg-Free	Serves 6	Prep time: 20 minutes	Cook time: 25 minutes

1 pound 80% to 90% percent lean ground beef

4 garlic cloves, minced

1 tablespoon dried oregano

¼ teaspoon kosher or sea salt

¼ teaspoon black pepper

½ cup part-skim ricotta cheese

1 (12-ounce) package wonton wrappers

1 (24-ounce) jar low-sodium tomato pasta sauce or 3 cups Easy Roasted Tomato Sauce (page 147)

The Italian American part of town in St. Louis, called The Hill, is where you can find the very best "toasted ravioli." This addicting appetizer of deep-fried meat-stuffed ravioli is a signature dish for the entire city. Here Serena found a way to make it an everyday Mediterranean dish—un-fried but still crispy and super dippable. Serve this as an appetizer or for dinner paired with our Kale Caesar Salad with Chickpeas (page 63) and crusty whole-grain bread. Make a vegetarian version of "t-ravs" by filling them with sautéed chopped mushrooms.

Preheat the oven to 375°F. Coat two large rimmed baking sheets with cooking spray.

Heat a skillet over medium-high heat and add the ground beef, garlic, oregano, salt, and black pepper. Cook, stirring frequently, until the beef is no longer pink, about 5 minutes. With a slotted spoon (to leave some of the fat behind in the pan), scoop out the beef mixture and place on a paper towel–covered plate to absorb more fat.

In a medium bowl, mix the cooked ground beef and ricotta cheese well.

Fill a small bowl with water and place it near your work surface. Place 1 wonton wrapper on a dry surface. (Keep the remaining wonton wrappers covered with a damp towel so they don't dry out.) Add 2 teaspoons of the beef filling to the center of the wrapper. Dip your finger in the water and run it along two sides of the wonton wrapper (to make the wrapper sticky). Fold the wonton wrapper over, matching two opposite corners to make a triangle; press the sides together to seal. Place the sealed ravioli on the baking sheet. Repeat with the remaining wonton wrappers, placing no more than 18 ravioli per baking sheet. (If the ravioli are crowded, they won't crisp in the oven.) Coat the tops of the ravioli with cooking spray. Place both baking sheets in the oven and cook for 10 minutes total, flipping the ravioli once after 5 minutes. Place the ravioli a serving platter.

continued

Crispy Ravioli with Tomato Dipping Sauce (continued)

While the first batch is cooking, make the rest of the ravioli with the remaining filling. Cook once the first batch comes out of the oven. When finished cooking, place the remaining ravioli on the serving platter and serve with the tomato sauce.

Healthy Kitchen Hack: Use wonton wrappers to make other easy snacks and meals. Some of our favorite "ravioli" fillings use just two ingredients: chopped cooked broccoli with shredded cheese; hummus with minced red bell peppers; ricotta cheese with tomato paste and fresh basil (okay, that's three ingredients, but you get the idea!).

Per Serving: Calories: 360; Total Fat: 10g; Saturated Fat: 4g; Cholesterol: 59mg; Sodium: 742mg; Total Carbohydrates: 43g; Fiber: 4g; Protein: 24g

Foolproof Pumpkin Gnocchi

Dairy-Free, Nut-Free, Vegetarian	Serves 6	Prep time: 20 minutes	Cook time: 15 minutes

1½ cups white whole-wheat flour, plus about 2 tablespoons more for rolling and drying

1 cup all-purpose flour

½ teaspoon ground nutmeg

2¼ teaspoons kosher or sea salt, divided

1 (15-ounce) can pumpkin puree

1 large egg yolk

1 (24-ounce) jar low-sodium tomato pasta sauce or 3 cups Easy Roasted Tomato Sauce (page 147)

Chopped fresh chives and grated Parmesan or Pecorino Romano cheese, for serving (optional)

Yes, you can make your own pillowy-soft gnocchi that's restaurant worthy! Serena had never made pasta from scratch before adapting Deanna's roasted butternut squash gnocchi recipe using canned pumpkin instead. But the process is simple, especially if you use a large stockpot for batch cooking. We make homemade pasta with primarily white whole-wheat flour because it resembles traditional semolina flour and the slightly coarse texture helps prevent the dough from sticking to your counter when shaping.

Sprinkle about 1 tablespoon white whole-wheat flour over two large rimmed baking sheets.

In a large bowl, whisk together the 1½ cups white whole-wheat flour with the all-purpose flour, nutmeg, and ¾ teaspoon of the salt. Add the pumpkin and egg yolk. Mix together with a fork. (The dough will be slightly sticky.) Divide the dough into four portions in the bowl. Remove the dough portions and add about 1 tablespoon white whole-wheat flour to the bowl. Add one portion of dough back into the bowl and coat with the flour. Using your hands on a well-floured surface, gently roll and pull the dough into a 16-inch-long log, about 1 inch in diameter. Cut the dough log into ¾-inch-long pieces and place each piece on the prepared baking sheet. Repeat with the three remaining dough portions.

Pour the pasta sauce into a medium saucepan and place on low heat to keep warm until serving time.

Place a large stockpot filled with water on the stove and cover. Bring to a boil and add the remaining 1½ teaspoons salt. Slide half of the gnocchi into the water. Boil until all the gnocchi rise to the top of the water, 4 to 5 minutes. Using a "kitchen spider" or slotted spoon, gently remove the gnocchi and place in the saucepan with the warmed pasta sauce. Repeat the boiling process with the remaining gnocchi.

continued

Foolproof Pumpkin Gnocchi (continued)

Serve the gnocchi in the pasta sauce and sprinkle with chives and Parmesan cheese, if desired.

Healthy Kitchen Hack: If not using right away, freeze your gnocchi to keep it fresh. Place your uncooked gnocchi on a large rimmed baking sheet lined with parchment paper. Place in the freezer until frozen, about 1 hour. Transfer the frozen gnocchi into zip-top plastic freezer bags. To cook from frozen, follow the instructions in the recipe and cook for about 5 to 6 minutes total before placing the gnocchi in the pasta sauce.

Per Serving: Calories: 259; Total Fat: 3g; Saturated Fat: 1g; Cholesterol: 31mg; Sodium: 586mg; Total Carbohydrates: 51g; Fiber: 8g; Protein: 9g

"This quick recipe makes an impressive homemade meal with common ingredients. I made it with my daughter-in-law long distance over Facebook Messenger and we felt so accomplished."

—Steph from Bridgeton, MO

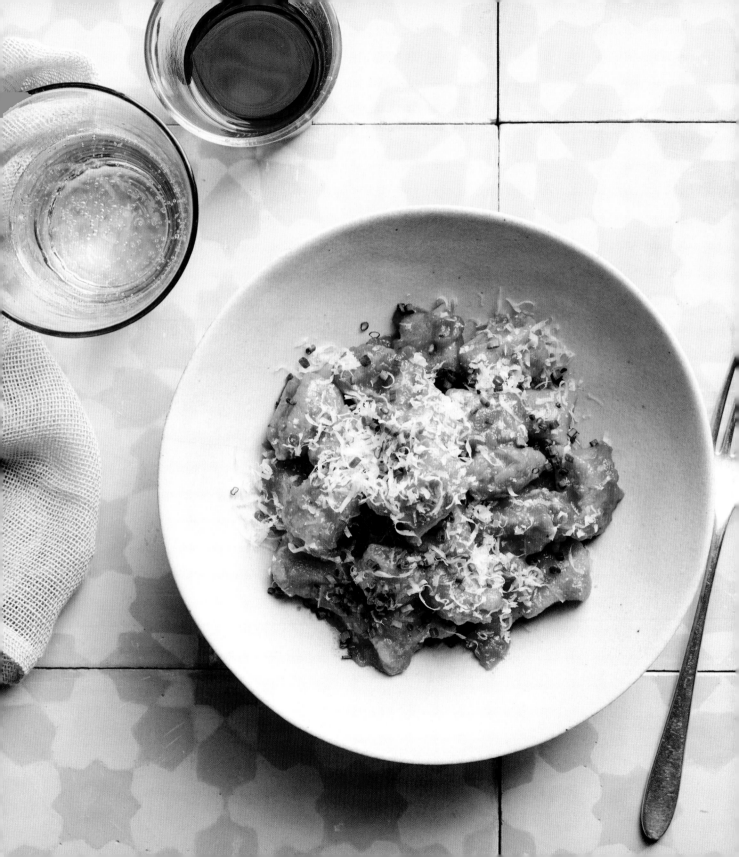

Baked Ziti with Sausage and Broccoli

Nut-Free, Egg-Free	Serves 8	Prep time: 10 minutes	Cook time: 20 minutes

1 head broccoli (1 pound)

¼ cup whole-wheat panko breadcrumbs

1 teaspoon extra-virgin olive oil

1½ teaspoons kosher or sea salt

1 (16-ounce) package ziti or penne pasta

8 ounces loose spicy Italian sausage

1 (24-ounces) jar low-sodium tomato pasta sauce

1 cup shredded part-skim mozzarella cheese (4 ounces)

Baked pasta dishes are hearty and comforting, but they can take at least 30 minutes to cook in the oven (and that's *after* you cook the pasta). With this recipe you'll be able to serve up a tomato sauce–laden noodle dish studded with spicy sausage and a golden cheese crust after only 5 minutes of oven time. (Our secret is to assemble all the ingredients warm in a large metal baking pan.) Bonus: The short baking time keeps the broccoli bright green.

Preheat the oven to 425°F. Place a 9×13-inch metal baking pan into the oven to warm.

Remove the little leaves from the broccoli stalks; chop and set aside. Chop the broccoli florets into bite-size pieces and set aside. Peel the tough skin off the broccoli stalks; slice the stalks into ¼-inch-thick coins and set aside.

In a small bowl, mix together the chopped broccoli leaves, breadcrumbs, and olive oil. Set aside.

Place a large stockpot filled with water on the stove and cover. Bring to a boil and add the salt. Add the pasta and stir. Cook the pasta according to the package directions until it is 1 minute short of al dente. Add the broccoli florets and stalk slices to the pot and cook until they just start to soften, about 3 minutes. Drain the pasta and broccoli, reserving ½ cup of the pasta water. Return the drained pasta, broccoli, and a few tablespoons of the pasta water to the stockpot.

While the pasta is cooking, place a medium skillet over medium-high heat. Cook the sausage, stirring frequently with a metal spatula or wooden spoon to break it up, until the meat is browned, 8 to 10 minutes. Add the pasta sauce and stir.

Remove the hot baking pan from the oven and carefully coat with cooking spray. Add the pasta-broccoli mix and the sausage sauce; mix gently. Sprinkle the cheese on top. Sprinkle the breadcrumb mixture over the cheese.

Bake for 5 minutes, until the cheese is melted and slightly golden.

Healthy Kitchen Hack: To save the step of peeling the broccoli stems, use broccolini (also called "baby broccoli") instead. The stems of this bright green vegetable are thin enough that they don't need peeling. A cross between broccoli and gai lan (Chinese broccoli), broccolini's flavor is on the sweeter side with a slight peppery edge. Just like broccoli, broccolini has the tiny stem leaves that are used here to brighten up the breadcrumb topping.

Per Serving: Calories: 407; Total Fat: 10g; Saturated Fat: 3g; Cholesterol: 30mg; Sodium: 283mg; Total Carbohydrates: 60g; Fiber: 6g; Protein: 18g

Kale and Chickpea Pappardelle

Dairy-Free, Nut-Free, Vegetarian	Serves 8	Prep time: 10 minutes	Cook time: 25 minutes

2 tablespoons extra-virgin olive oil

1 medium onion, chopped (about 2 cups)

2 garlic cloves, minced

1½ teaspoons ground cumin

½ teaspoon black pepper

3 cups chopped kale leaves and stems

½ cup golden raisins

1 medium orange

1¾ teaspoons kosher or sea salt, divided

1 (16-ounce) package pappardelle or fettuccine

1 (15-ounce) can chickpeas, drained and rinsed, liquid reserved

2 tablespoons sesame seeds

This colorful pasta is now one of Serena's children's favorite dishes, but before the kids tasted it, the announcement that kale was part of dinner was not met with happy cheers. If you also don't applaud for kale, please give this pasta a chance. We pair it with sunny Mediterranean ingredients like sweet golden raisins, acidic orange juice, crunchy sesame seeds, and nutty chickpeas. Plus, there's a secret ingredient to help coat the thick pappardelle noodles in an extra-creamy yet dairy-free sauce. (See the Healthy Kitchen Hack opposite.)

Heat the oil in a large skillet over medium heat. Add the onion and cook, stirring occasionally, until just golden, 8 to 10 minutes. Push the onion mixture to the sides of the skillet and add the garlic, cumin, and black pepper. Cook, stirring constantly, for 1 minute. Add the kale and raisins and cook, stirring occasionally, for 10 minutes. During the last few minutes of cooking, grate the orange zest with a Microplane or citrus zester over the kale and stir well. Cut the orange in half and squeeze the juice from both halves into a small bowl. Set aside.

While the onions and kale cook, place a large stockpot filled with water over high heat. Bring to a boil and add 1½ teaspoons of the salt. Add the pasta and stir. Cook according to the package instructions until about 1 minute shy of al dente. Drain the pasta, reserving 1 cup of the pasta water; add the pasta back to the stockpot along with the chickpeas and ¼ cup of the pasta water.

Once the kale has cooked for 10 minutes, add the remaining ¼ teaspoon salt, ¾ cup of the reserved chickpea liquid, and ¼ cup of the pasta water to the skillet. Cook, stirring occasionally, until the sauce turns creamy, about 2 minutes. Add as much of the pasta as will fit in the skillet and toss to combine.

To a serving bowl, add the pasta-kale mixture from the skillet, any remaining pasta in the stockpot, the orange juice, and the sesame seeds; toss to combine, then serve.

Healthy Kitchen Hack: Have you heard about aquafaba? It's the liquid in canned chickpeas and it helps make this pasta sauce creamy without any dairy. Because aquafaba is so starchy, it can be used as a thickener and even as an egg replacement. It whips up into a frothy foam and is what makes our hummus (on page 50) so light and airy.

Per Serving: Calories: 365; Total Fat: 7g; Saturated Fat: 1g; Cholesterol: 0mg; Sodium: 286mg; Total Carbohydrates: 66g; Fiber: 6g; Protein: 12g

Ricotta-Walnut Spaghetti and Zucchini Noodles

Egg-Free, Vegetarian | Serves 6 | Prep time: 10 minutes | Cook time: 25 minutes

⅔ cup walnut pieces

1¾ teaspoons kosher or sea salt, divided

8 ounces dried spaghetti

⅓ cup sun-dried tomatoes (dry from a pouch), thinly sliced (about 1 ounce)

2 medium or 3 small zucchini (10 to 12 ounces total)

3 tablespoons extra-virgin olive oil, divided

2 garlic cloves, minced

¼ teaspoon crushed red pepper

½ cup part-skim ricotta cheese

2 tablespoons grated Parmesan or Pecorino Romano cheese

¼ teaspoon black pepper

This tempting dish is a great way to introduce the idea of vegetable noodles to first-timers by mixing them with everyone's favorite: spaghetti. While zucchini noodles—or zoodles—are the most popular veggie to spiralize (and the mildest in flavor), you can also swap in carrots, sweet potatoes, or beets to add color and distinct flavors. Deanna likes to add canned tuna to this dish make a modern version of her favorite dinner from the '70s: tuna noodle casserole.

Place a large skillet over medium heat. Toss in the walnuts and cook, stirring occasionally, until they are lightly toasted, 4 to 6 minutes. Set aside and wipe the skillet clean with a towel.

Place a large stockpot filled with water on the stove and cover. Bring to a boil and add 1½ teaspoons of the salt. Add the spaghetti and stir. Cook according to the package instructions. Once the water returns to a boil, remove ½ cup of the pasta water and pour it into a small bowl with the sun-dried tomatoes. Set aside. When the pasta is done cooking, drain it, reserving ½ to ¾ cup of the pasta water.

While the pasta cooks, make the zucchini noodles using a spiralizer or a box grater. (See the Healthy Kitchen Hack opposite.) Add the zucchini to a bowl with 2 tablespoons of the olive oil and the remaining ¼ teaspoon salt; toss until coated.

Return the skillet to medium heat and pour in the remaining 1 tablespoon olive oil. Add the garlic and crushed red pepper. Cook, stirring constantly, for 30 seconds. Add the zucchini and toss until coated with the seasonings. Cook for 2 minutes, then add 3 to 4 tablespoons of the pasta water.

Add the drained spaghetti to the skillet and toss with the zucchini noodles. Heat together for another minute, adding a few more tablespoons of the pasta water if needed to prevent everything from sticking together.

Into a large serving bowl, put the ricotta cheese, Parmesan cheese, and black pepper. Whisk in about 3 tablespoons of the pasta water and 3 tablespoons of the soaking water from the sun-dried tomatoes to make a creamy sauce. Add the cooked spaghetti and zucchini and the toasted walnuts. Drain the sun-dried tomatoes and add them to the bowl. Toss all the ingredients together until well coated. Serve immediately.

Healthy Kitchen Hack: Zucchini noodles are easiest to make with a tabletop or handheld spiralizer but if you don't want to purchase another gadget for your kitchen, there are other options. Take a vegetable peeler or a mandoline slicer and carefully run the long side of the zucchini against the blade to create wide and long noodle shapes. Stack the noodles and cut them lengthwise into thin noodles. Or take your box grater and hold it at a 45-degree angle with largest grater holes facing up. Run the long side of the zucchini down the grater in slow, long strokes to create "zoodles."

Per Serving: Calories: 353; Total Fat: 19g; Saturated Fat: 3g; Cholesterol: 8mg; Sodium: 174mg; Total Carbohydrates: 38g; Fiber: 4g; Protein: 12g

"I loved the combo of zucchini and pasta. The sun-dried tomatoes added a lot of flavor and I liked it with an extra hit of crushed red pepper. I would make this again!"

—Lenna from Langley, WA

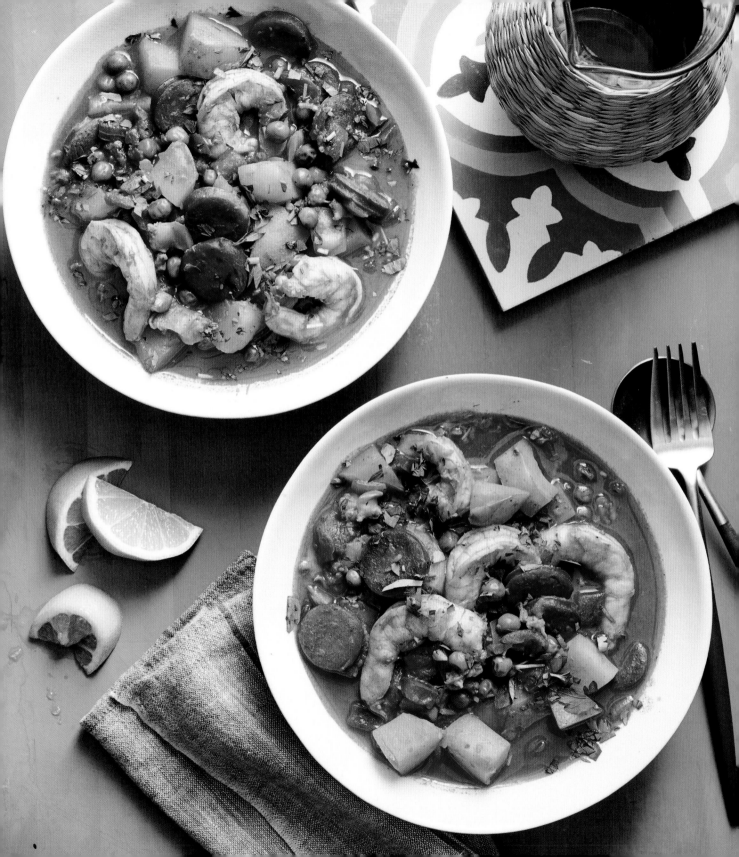

seafood

Microwave Salmon with Green Onions

Dairy-Free, Nut-Free, Gluten-Free, Egg-Free	Serves 2	Prep time: 5 minutes	Cook time: 5 minutes

6 green onions

2 (4-ounce) boneless salmon fillets, skin-on or skinless

1 medium lemon, cut in half

1 tablespoon extra-virgin olive oil

⅛ teaspoon kosher or sea salt

Many people need a little encouragement to eat more seafood and here's some to get you started: Microwave fish dinners can be on the table in less than 10 minutes. Microwaving almost any type of fish is probably our favorite way to cook fillets, because it's really hard to overcook the fish using this method. And even if someone is late to dinner, it can be made to order.

Coat a glass pie dish or large low-sided microwave-safe bowl with cooking spray.

Cut the green onions in half. Lay them on the bottom of the prepared pie dish. Top with the salmon fillets, skin-side down if they have skin. If the fillets have an end that is thinner, fold that end under so that the fillet is roughly the same thickness throughout.

Squeeze 1 tablespoon of lemon juice into a small bowl. (Save any remaining lemon for another use.) Add the olive oil and salt, then whisk together. Pour over both pieces of salmon. Cover the dish with plastic wrap, leaving a small hole at the edge to vent the steam.

Microwave on high for 2 minutes. Carefully remove the hot dish and let some of the steam escape before opening the plastic wrap. Check the doneness by using a fork to see if the fish is just starting to separate into flakes. If any part of the fillet doesn't look cooked, microwave, covered with plastic wrap as before, in 20-second increments until done. (For reference, fillets that are about ¾ inch thick do not need more than 3 minutes of cooking time.)

Serve the fish and green onions with the sauce from the bottom of the cooking dish.

Per Serving: Calories: 205; Total Fat: 12g; Saturated Fat: 2g; Cholesterol: 52mg; Sodium: 204mg; Total Carbohydrates: 3g; Fiber: 1g; Protein: 23g

Healthy Kitchen Hack: For a quick side that's finished at the same time as the fish, add 1 cup of shredded cabbage per fillet to the bottom of the dish before cooking. Lay the green onions on top and then the fish. Cook as above, but the total cooking time for both the cabbage and fish will be 3 to 4 minutes instead of 2 to 3 minutes.

Tuna Niçoise for Two

| Dairy-Free, Nut-Free, Gluten-Free | Serves 2 | Prep time: 5 minutes | Cook time: 5 minutes |

4 small (2-inch diameter) Yukon Gold potatoes (about 8 ounces)

¼ cup canned or jarred olives any variety, 2 tablespoons of the can/jar liquid, reserved separately, divided

1 cup frozen whole green beans

1 medium lemon, cut in half

1 teaspoon dried crushed oregano leaves

¼ teaspoon freshly ground black pepper

1 (5-ounce) can tuna in olive oil

½ English cucumber, sliced

2 hard-boiled large eggs (see the Healthy Kitchen Hack on page 117), peeled and halved

If you have 10 minutes to spare in the morning, you can pack this tangy, protein-packed tuna salad for lunch (and store the other half in the fridge for lunch the next day). Or you can easily double this salad to serve four and enjoy it, perhaps with a glass of white wine, as a light and more relaxed dinner meal.

Slice the potatoes in half and place on a large microwave-safe plate. Drizzle 1 tablespoon of the olive liquid and 1 tablespoon water over them. Cover with a paper towel and microwave on high, stirring halfway through, for about 4 minutes, until the potatoes have just softened. Place the potatoes into two individual salad bowls or (if you're packing lunches) two to-go containers. On the same plate, place the green beans and cover. Microwave for 1 minute on defrost. Top the potatoes with the beans.

Squeeze 2 tablespoons of lemon juice into a medium bowl. (Save any remaining lemon for another use.) Add the remaining 1 tablespoon olive liquid, the oregano, and the black pepper. Using a fork, lift the tuna out of the can, letting most of the oil drain away, and add it to the lemon juice mixture. Toss gently. Divide the tuna between the two bowls. Top with the cucumbers, olives, and eggs.

Healthy Kitchen Hack: Even if you don't have any lettuce in your refrigerator, you can still have salad. Frozen vegetables can fill your plate with produce any time of year. The key is to make these veggies taste as close to fresh as possible, which usually means thawing them gently. Thaw frozen peas, corn, beans, cauliflower, and broccoli in the fridge overnight. Then add your other salad ingredients, toss with your favorite dressing, and eat chilled.

Per Serving: Calories: 317; Total Fat: 11g; Saturated Fat: 2g; Cholesterol: 209mg; Sodium: 835mg; Total Carbohydrates: 31g; Fiber: 5g; Protein: 27g

Baked Salmon with Creamy Cilantro Sauce

| Nut-Free, Gluten-Free, Egg-Free | Serves 4 | Prep time: 10 minutes | Cook time: 25 minutes |

1 pound skinless salmon fillet (about 1 inch thick)

2 teaspoons extra-virgin olive oil

½ teaspoon kosher or sea salt, divided

¼ teaspoon black pepper

1 medium lemon, cut in half

½ cup fresh cilantro

⅓ cup plain 2% Greek yogurt

1 garlic clove

¾ teaspoon honey

½ teaspoon ground cumin

Omega-3 fatty acids—most commonly found in fatty fish like salmon—play a crucial role in supporting brain function and memory. And while you won't find many species of salmon swimming in the Mediterranean Sea, salmon contains a high concentration of these heart-healthy fats that are an essential part of the Mediterranean Diet. Plus, it's a variety of fish commonly enjoyed and available Stateside. Pair this simple yet special dish with our Orange, Celery, and Olive Tabbouleh (page 66) or our Charred Green Beans with Za'atar (page 76).

Preheat the oven to 375°F. Let the salmon sit at room temperature for 10 minutes.

Cut a piece of aluminum foil approximately twice the length of the salmon and place it on a large rimmed baking sheet. Place the salmon on one half of the foil. If one side of the salmon is thinner, tuck that side under so the fillet is approximately the same thickness. Brush the top of the salmon with the olive oil and season with ¼ teaspoon of the salt and the black pepper. Thinly slice one half of the lemon and place the slices on top of the salmon. Reserve the other lemon half.

Fold the foil over the salmon and tightly crimp the edges to seal. Bake for 22 to 25 minutes or until the salmon just barely starts to flake in the thickest part. Remove from the oven and carefully open the foil to let the steam out. Using a spatula, transfer the salmon to a serving plate and transfer the lemon slices to a small plate for serving.

While the salmon is cooking, squeeze 1 tablespoon of juice from the reserved lemon half into a blender or food processor. (Save any remaining lemon for another use.) Add 1 tablespoon water and the cilantro, yogurt, garlic, honey, cumin, and remaining ¼ teaspoon salt. Process until smooth.

Drizzle half of the cilantro-yogurt sauce over the salmon. Serve the extra sauce in a small bowl. Serve the lemon slices for squeezing over the salmon, if desired.

Healthy Kitchen Hack: Switch up this sauce by swapping in different herb-and-spice combinations for the cilantro and cumin; try fresh parsley with grated lemon zest, fresh dill with chives, or fresh mint with a dash of crushed red pepper.

Per Serving: Calories: 207; Total Fat: 10g; Saturated Fat: 2g; Cholesterol: 53mg; Sodium: 300mg; Total Carbohydrates: 3g; Fiber: 0g; Protein: 27g

"This salmon was a huge dinner success—
my whole family loved it and also
appreciated the easy cleanup!"

—Allison from Plymouth, MI

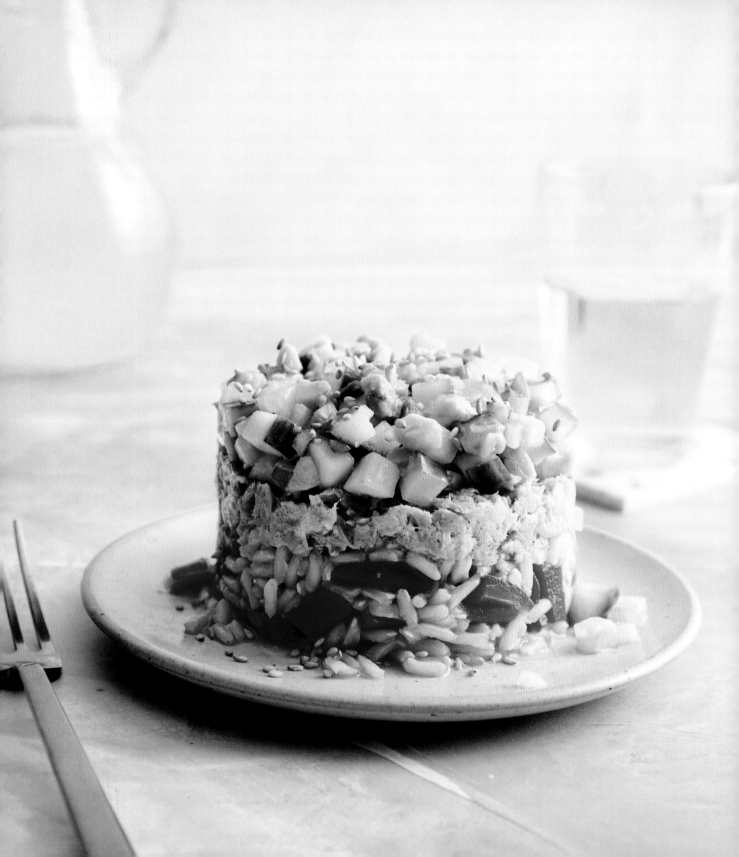

Tuna Basmati Rice Stacks

Nut-Free, Gluten-Free, Egg-Free	Serves 4	Prep time: 15 minutes

1 medium lime

2½ cups cooked brown basmati rice

1 (12-ounce) jar roasted red peppers or 2 Roasted Red Peppers (page 44), drained and chopped

2 (5-ounce) cans tuna in olive oil, undrained

¼ cup plain 2% Greek yogurt (about 4 ounces)

½ tablespoon extra-virgin olive oil

¼ teaspoon za'atar (or dried thyme)

⅛ teaspoon kosher or sea salt

1 avocado, pitted and diced

1 large cucumber, diced

¼ cup minced red onion

⅛ teaspoon crushed red pepper

1 teaspoon sesame seeds

Inspired by sushi rice stacks, Deanna applied Mediterranean ingredients to this fun-to-assemble and easy-to-make meal. The leftovers are just as good and you can turn this recipe into tuna burgers, too (see the Healthy Kitchen Hack below). Any type of rice (preferably brown) will work here. To cut cooking time, try instant brown or frozen cooked brown rice.

Squeeze 1 tablespoon of lime juice into a large bowl. (Reserve the remaining lime.) Add the cooked rice and roasted peppers. Mix well and set aside.

In another bowl, mix the tuna, yogurt, olive oil, za'atar, and salt and set aside.

Into a third bowl, squeeze another 1 tablespoon of lime juice. (Save any remaining lime for another use.) Add the avocado, cucumber, onion, and crushed red pepper. Mix well and set aside.

To form the tuna stacks, use a 1-cup measuring cup coated with cooking spray. Place one-fourth of the avocado mixture on the bottom of the measuring cup. Layer with one-fourth of the tuna mixture and top with one-fourth of the rice mixture. Place a plate upside down on top of the measuring cup and flip it over. Carefully lift up the measuring cup, leaving the stack behind on the plate. Sprinkle with ¼ teaspoon of the sesame seeds. Repeat with the remaining ingredients to make four stacks in total.

Healthy Kitchen Hack: Use this recipe to make tuna rice burgers! In a large bowl, combine the red pepper rice mixture with the tuna mixture. For every 1 cup in the bowl, add 1 egg (to help bind the patties). Mix well. Form ⅓ cup of mixture into 3-inch patties. Cook in a medium skillet coated with cooking spray over medium heat for 5 minutes. Carefully flip and cook for another 5 minutes. Top with sesame seeds and serve with the avocado mixture.

Per Serving: Calories: 388; Total Fat: 13g; Saturated Fat: 1g; Cholesterol: 24mg; Sodium: 580mg; Total Carbohydrates: 49g; Fiber: 5g; Protein: 23g

Skillet Shrimp with Tomatoes and Feta

Nut-Free, Gluten-Free, Egg-Free	Serves 6	Prep time: 10 minutes	Cook time: 10 minutes

2 tablespoons extra-virgin olive oil

2 garlic cloves, minced

¼ teaspoon crushed red pepper

2 large tomatoes, chopped, or 1 quart grape tomatoes, cut in half (about 3 cups)

1 (14.5-ounce) can low-sodium diced tomatoes

1 teaspoon dried oregano

¼ teaspoon kosher or sea salt

¼ teaspoon black pepper

1½ pounds frozen medium shrimp, thawed, peeled, and tails removed

1 (8-ounce) block feta cheese, at room temperature

⅓ cup chopped fresh parsley

Every time Deanna visits her aunt and uncle on Whidbey Island, Washington, she comes home with oodles of recipe inspiration. Aunt Lenna is a fantastic cook and can always whip up an incredible appetizer for the party boat (they live on a lake). She served this Mediterranean-esque one right from the skillet along with warmed pita for sopping up the amazing sauce.

In a large skillet over medium heat, heat the olive oil for 1 minute. Add the garlic and crushed red pepper and cook, stirring frequently, for 30 seconds. Add the chopped tomatoes, canned tomatoes, oregano, salt, and black pepper. Turn up the heat to medium-high and cook, stirring frequently, for 2 minutes to bring the ingredients to a simmer.

Reduce the heat to medium and push down on the tomatoes with a wooden spoon to break them open further. Add the shrimp and stir. With the spoon, clear an area in the center of the sauce and add the feta. Cook the shrimp and feta, stirring the shrimp a few times carefully around the feta (to keep the cheese block intact) until the shrimp are cooked through and have just turned pink, 5 to 6 minutes. Remove the skillet from the heat and break up the feta with a serving spoon. Top with the parsley and serve.

Healthy Kitchen Hack: Swap out the shrimp for salmon, tuna, or cod fillets, cover and cook for 10 to 12 minutes, until they just start to flake or measure 145°F on a meat thermometer. Thinner fish like tilapia, flounder, and rainbow trout will cook quicker, closer to 8 to 10 minutes. Add the feta for the last 5 minutes of cooking.

Per Serving: Calories: 271; Total Fat: 11g; Saturated Fat: 6g; Cholesterol: 216mg; Sodium: 678mg; Total Carbohydrates: 12g; Fiber: 2g; Protein: 31g

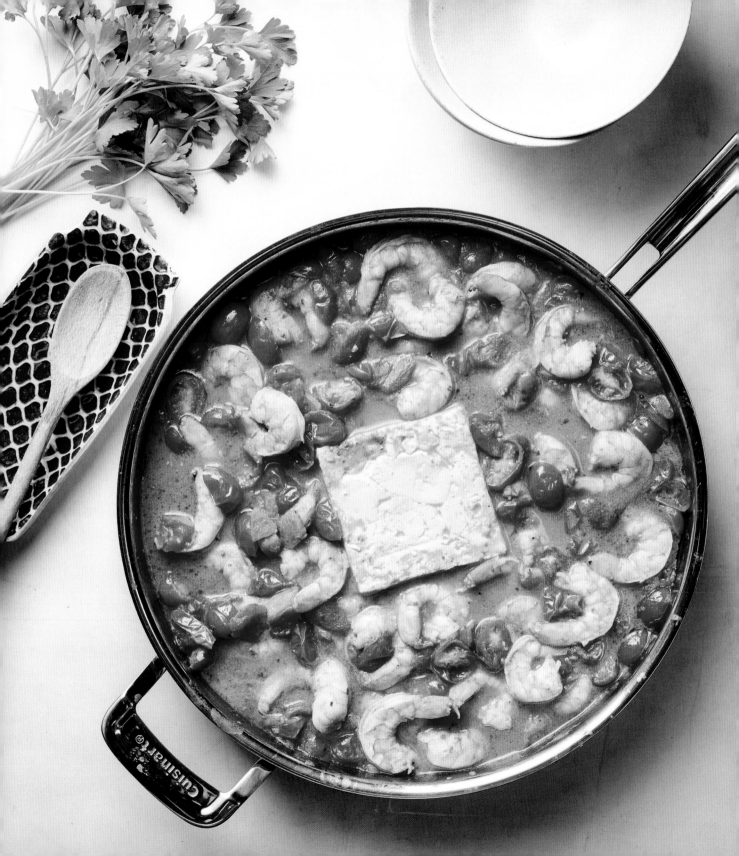

Simple Salmon Kebabs

Dairy-Free, Nut-Free, Gluten-Free, Egg-Free	Serves 4	Prep time: 15 minutes	Cook time: 15 minutes

1 pound skinless salmon fillet

1 head broccoli with stem (about ½ pound)

8 mini sweet peppers

1 pint grape tomatoes

¼ teaspoon kosher or sea salt

Cilantro-Olive Salsa (page 79) or topping sauce of your choice, or Spicy Sweet Quick Pickles (page 51), for serving

Grab a pound of salmon—or any type of fish—with any veggies you have hanging around and make this "no rotating required" dinner-on-a-stick. We like to serve these kebabs with the Cilantro-Olive Salsa from our Roasted Butternut Squash but you can serve with any condiment like pesto, tomato salsa, ketchup—or the only topping that will get all Serena's kids to eat fish: dill pickles.

Preheat the oven to 425°F. Line two large rimmed baking sheets with parchment paper.

Cut the fish into 1½-inch squares. (See the Healthy Kitchen Hack below.)

Cut the broccoli into 1-inch florets. Slice off any tough peel on the broccoli stalk, then slice the stalk into ½-inch rounds. Set aside.

Sort the mini peppers into two piles: ones that longer than 2 inches and ones that are 2 inches or shorter. Leave the shorter peppers whole. Slice the longer ones in half from stem end to bottom. Scrape out the seeds but keep the stems intact.

Using 8 metal or 12 wooden skewers (no need to soak wooden skewers), thread the fish, broccoli, mini peppers, and tomatoes, leaving about ½ inch between each piece. Place the kebabs on the prepared baking sheets. Coat the tops of the fish and vegetables with cooking spray. Sprinkle with the salt.

Bake for 10 to 12 minutes or until the fish just barely starts to flake and the broccoli just starts to singe on the edges. Serve the kebabs with the sauce of your choice or pickles.

Healthy Kitchen Hack: To ensure even cooking, cut the fish into uniform pieces.

Per Serving (without sauce): Calories: 207; Total Fat: 6g; Saturated Fat: 1g; Cholesterol: 58mg; Sodium: 234mg; Total Carbohydrates: 12g; Fiber: 4g; Protein: 28g

Crunchy Salmon Nuggets

Nut-Free		Serves 4	Prep time: 15 minutes	Cook time: 10 minutes

1 medium lemon

2 (5-ounce) cans skinless, boneless salmon, drained

⅔ cup panko breadcrumbs, divided

¼ cup plain 2% Greek yogurt

¼ cup crumbled feta cheese (1 ounce)

1 large egg

½ teaspoon garlic powder

½ teaspoon black pepper

Olive Oil–Yogurt Spread (page 42), for serving (optional)

These little nuggets of flavor will have kids and adults eating their recommended two servings of seafood a week. Serena served them for the first time when her daughter was studying for her high school algebra final. Maybe it was because they are packed with omega-3s for extra brain power, but she aced her final! Whip them up into "cute" little nuggets or shape them into four larger salmon burgers.

Preheat the oven to 425°F. Place a large rimmed baking sheet in the oven to heat.

Using a Microplane or citrus zester, grate the lemon zest into a large bowl. Cut the lemon in half and squeeze 2 tablespoons of the juice into the bowl. Slice the partially squeezed lemon halves into wedges and set aside for serving with the finished nuggets.

Add the salmon to the bowl and, using a fork, mash into fine flakes. Add ⅓ cup of the panko along with the yogurt, feta, egg, garlic powder, and black pepper. Mix well to combine.

Using a 1-tablespoon measuring spoon, scoop portions of the salmon mixture onto a large plate. Sprinkle the top of each with about 2½ table-spoons (total) of the panko, pressing gently so the crumbs adhere to the salmon nuggets.

Carefully remove the hot baking sheet from the oven and coat with cooking spray. Transfer the nuggets, crumb-side down, onto the hot pan. Sprinkle the remaining panko on top of the nuggets, pressing to adhere. (It's fine if some crumbs fall onto the baking sheet.)

Bake for 5 minutes. Remove the baking sheet from the oven and flip the nuggets using a thin metal spatula. Bake for 5 more minutes. Serve with the lemon wedges and Olive Oil–Yogurt Spread, if desired.

continued

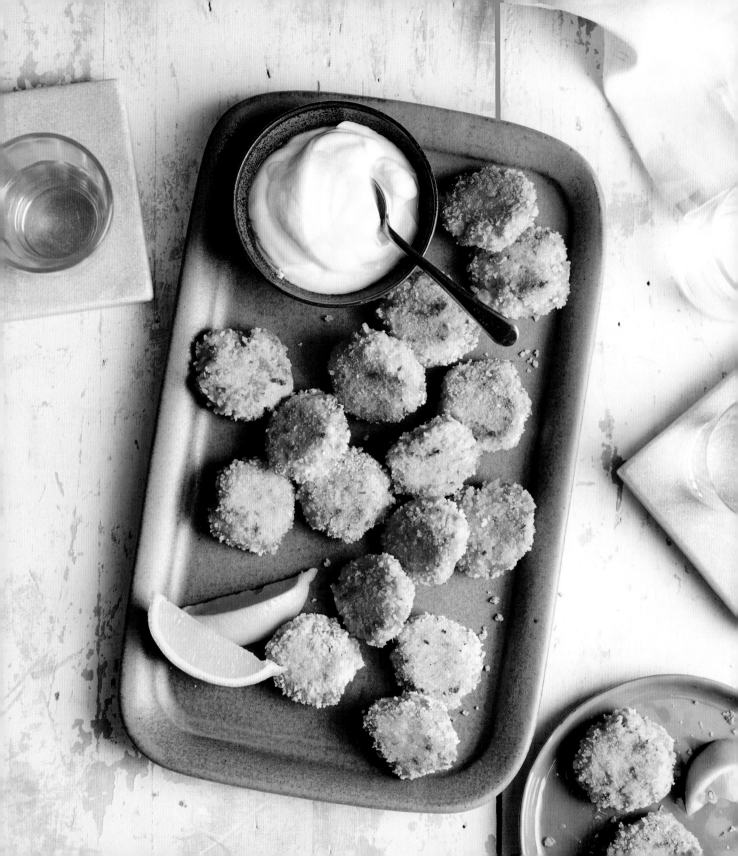

Healthy Kitchen Hack: Canned salmon is an often-overlooked staple in the Mediterranean pantry. It doesn't have to be thawed like frozen salmon or used up quickly like fresh fish from the fish counter. With this recipe, we also tested two 7-ounce cans of bone-in, skin-on salmon and they worked deliciously. The bones add extra calcium and are easily mashed into the salmon mixture, as is the omega-3-rich salmon skin.

Per Serving: Calories: 178; Total Fat: 6g; Saturated Fat: 3g; Cholesterol: 84mg; Sodium: 300mg; Total Carbohydrates: 13g; Fiber: 1g; Protein: 17g

Manhattan Paella

Dairy-Free, Nut-Free, Gluten-Free, Egg-Free	Serves 6	Prep time: 10 minutes	Cook time: 30 minutes

1 tablespoon extra-virgin olive oil

1 cup chopped onion (about ½ medium onion)

1 large green bell pepper, chopped

1 teaspoon ground turmeric

1 teaspoon sweet paprika

2 links Spanish chorizo sausage (about 8 ounces) or kielbasa, cut into ¼-inch pieces

3 garlic cloves, minced

6 small Yukon Gold potatoes (about 1 pound), cut into ¾-inch cubes

1 (15-ounce) can low-sodium diced tomatoes

2 cups low-sodium chicken broth

1 (10-ounce) can baby clams

½ pound frozen uncooked medium shrimp, thawed, peeled, and tails removed

1 cup frozen green peas

1 cup chopped fresh parsley

1 medium lemon, sliced into wedges, for serving

This comforting dish is chock-full of the tantalizing ingredients found in *both* Manhattan clam chowder and Spanish paella, without the rice, but with the spicy chorizo sausage! During recipe testing, Serena served it to some unexpected dinner guests and as a last-minute inspiration, she served it with corn tortilla chips, which ended up being the perfect quick accompaniment. By the way, this is hands-down her favorite recipe in the book.

In a large stockpot over medium-high heat, heat the olive oil. Add the onion, green pepper, turmeric, and paprika and cook, stirring occasionally, for 8 minutes. Using a long spoon, push the onion mixture to the sides of the pot, add the sausage, and cook, stirring occasionally, until the sausage is browned, about 3 minutes. Push the sausage to the side of the pot and add the garlic; cook, stirring constantly, for 1 minute. Add the potatoes, tomatoes, broth, and 1 cup water. Using a slotted spoon, strain the clams over the pot so only the liquid from the can is added. Increase the heat to high and bring to a boil. Reduce the heat to medium and cook until the potatoes are just soft when tested with a fork, about 8 minutes. Add the clams, shrimp, and peas. Cook until the shrimp just turn pink, 2 to 4 minutes; don't overcook. Stir in the parsley and serve with the lemon wedges.

Healthy Kitchen Hack: Make this dish, and any of our shrimp recipes, more budget-friendly with shell-on (deveined) uncooked frozen shrimp. Cooking shrimp in the shell protects it from overcooking and becoming tough, and maintains the delicate flavor. Eating with your hands is usually synonymous with *really* good food, so just add a small plate to each place setting for discarded shells.

Per Serving: Calories: 315; Total Fat: 12g; Saturated Fat: 4g; Cholesterol: 89mg; Sodium: 866mg; Total Carbohydrates: 30g; Fiber: 6g; Protein: 23g

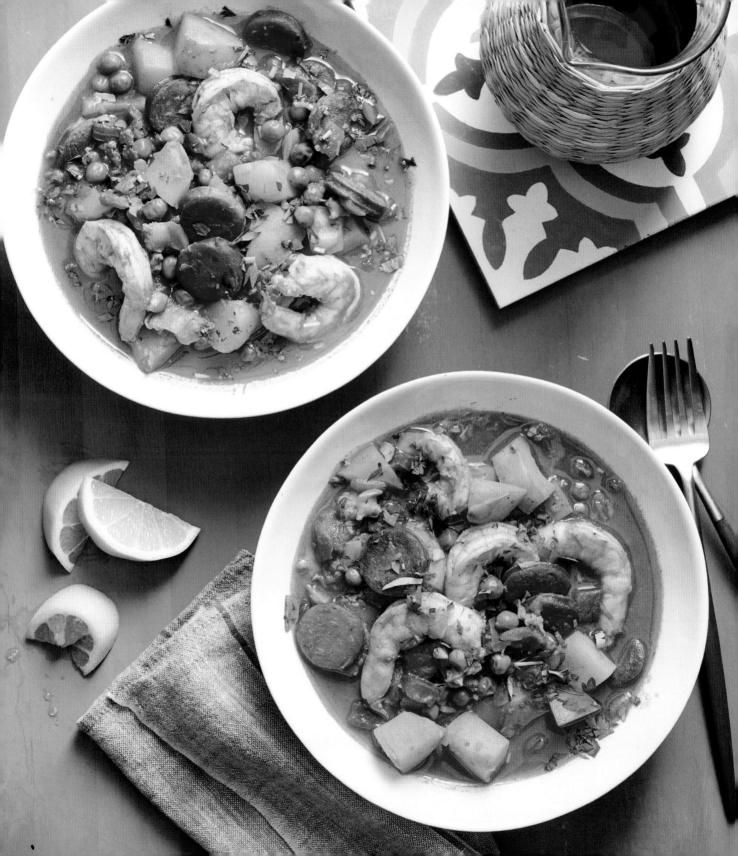

Rosemary Shrimp with Sweet Potato Polenta

| Nut-Free, Gluten-Free, Egg-Free | Serves 4 | Prep time: 15 minutes | Cook time: 20 minutes |

1 pound frozen uncooked large shrimp, thawed, peeled, and tails removed

2 tablespoons extra-virgin olive oil

2 garlic cloves, minced

1 tablespoon chopped fresh rosemary or 1 teaspoon dried

1 tablespoon chopped fresh thyme or 1 teaspoon dried

¼ teaspoon black pepper

1 large sweet potato

2 (18-ounce) tubes plain polenta

1½ cups reduced-fat (2%) milk

3 tablespoons grated Parmesan or Pecorino Romano cheese

Every year on Christmas Eve, Deanna makes a version of this aromatic shrimp for her Italian American family's traditional Seven-Fish Dinner. But it's actually simple enough to make for weeknight meals. In this recipe, we serve the shrimp with a hearty portion of cheesy sweet potato–enriched polenta. If you're making this for company, thread the uncooked shrimp on fresh rosemary sprigs, cook about 3 minutes per side, and serve the mini "skewers" on top of each bowl of polenta.

Into a large bowl, put the shrimp, olive oil, garlic, rosemary, thyme, and black pepper. Using tongs or your hands, mix all the ingredients together until the shrimp is evenly coated. Set aside.

Using a fork, poke several holes in the sweet potato to allow steam to escape. Place on a microwave-safe plate and microwave on high for 8 to 10 minutes, until the flesh is completely soft. Using oven mitts, remove from the microwave and cool slightly. Scoop the flesh into a bowl and mash with a potato masher or a fork. Set aside.

While the sweet potato is cooking, place a large skillet over medium-high heat. Add the shrimp and its marinade and cook, stirring occasionally, until the shrimp just turn pink, 5 to 6 minutes. Remove from the heat to prevent overcooking.

To heat up the polenta, remove the plastic wrap from around the tube. Slice one tube of the polenta into ½-inch-thick thick rounds and place in a microwave-safe bowl. Microwave on high for 1 minute. Place the heated polenta in a large stockpot. Repeat the slicing and heating process with the remaining tube of polenta, then add that to the pot. Mash the heated polenta with a potato masher or fork until coarsely mashed.

Place the pot with the polenta over medium heat. Add the milk and whisk until completely absorbed. Add the mashed sweet potato to the pot and whisk it into the polenta until smooth. Continue to heat the polenta until warm, 2 to 3 more minutes. Remove from the heat and stir in the Parmesan cheese until melted. Divide among four bowls, top with the cooked shrimp, and serve.

Healthy Kitchen Hack: If you can't find tubed polenta, making it from scratch is simple (as we do with our Cream of Polenta with Pears and Walnuts on page 27). Start with 1 cup cornmeal (fine-, medium-, or coarsely-ground) and 4 cups of your choice of liquid. Water is typically used as it lets the corn flavor shine through, but we also like to use milk for creaminess or broth to add extra flavor. In a medium saucepan, whisk together the cornmeal and liquid. Over medium-high heat, bring the mixture to a simmer, whisking occasionally. Reduce the heat to medium-low and cook, stirring frequently, until the polenta thickens, about 15 minutes. (If you prefer a sweeter, stronger corn flavor, cook for another 10 to 15 minutes.)

Per Serving: Calories 400; Total Fat: 11g; Saturated Fat: 3g; Cholesterol: 193mg; Sodium: 786mg; Total Carbohydrates: 47g; Fiber: 9g; Protein: 30g

Pistachio-Parmesan Crusted Cod

Egg-Free		Serves 4	Prep time: 10 minutes	Cook time: 15 minutes

½ cup shelled pistachios

⅓ cup panko breadcrumbs

2 tablespoons grated Parmesan or Pecorino Romano cheese

⅓ cup plain 2% Greek yogurt

1 pound cod fillet or other firm white fish, cut into 4 pieces

½ teaspoon kosher or sea salt, divided

½ teaspoon black pepper, divided

1 (15-ounce) can mandarin oranges in light syrup

2 tablespoons extra-virgin olive oil

1 teaspoon honey

1 teaspoon Dijon mustard

2½ cups arugula or spinach leaves

If people you cook for say they don't like fish but love nuts (or maybe this is you?), this is the recipe to change minds. The pistachio-and-Parmesan coating provides an appealing crispy texture and a slightly addicting flavor that will have anyone coming back for seconds. Pistachios are a quintessential nut found in both sweet and savory Mediterranean recipes, but you can swap them out for almonds, walnuts, or pecans, if you prefer.

Preheat the oven to 400°F. Place a wire rack over a large rimmed baking sheet and coat both with cooking spray.

Put the pistachios into a food processor. Pulse several times until the nuts resemble the texture of breadcrumbs. In a large bowl, mix together the chopped pistachios with the breadcrumbs and Parmesan cheese. Set aside.

Into another large bowl, put the yogurt and 2 tablespoons water. Whisk together to thin out the yogurt. Set aside.

Pat dry the fish fillets with a paper towel. Sprinkle ¼ teaspoon of the salt and ¼ teaspoon of the black pepper over both sides of all the fillets. Dip one fillet in the yogurt mixture and coat it on both sides. Slide any excess yogurt back into the bowl with your hands. Dip the yogurt-covered fillet into the pistachio-Parmesan coating, turning to make sure both sides are fully covered. Place the coated fillet on the prepared rack and repeat the coating process with the remaining fillets. Discard any extra coating or yogurt.

Bake the fish for 10 to 15 minutes, until the thickest fillet just starts to flake in the middle. (The cooking time will vary based on the thickness of the fillets.)

While the fish cooks, drain the mandarin oranges through a strainer over a bowl to save some of the liquid. Add 1 tablespoon of the liquid to a small bowl along with the olive oil, honey, mustard, remaining ¼ teaspoon salt, and remaining ¼ teaspoon black pepper. Whisk together to make a dressing.

Place the arugula on one part of a large serving platter; add the mandarin oranges. Drizzle with the dressing and toss to coat. Place the cooked cod fillets next to the arugula salad and serve.

Healthy Kitchen Hack: If you don't have a food processor, manually chopping nuts, like pistachios, can be tricky because they roll around. So, try our "smacking" method instead. Add the nuts to a large zip-top plastic bag and seal. With a rolling pin, a small skillet, or the back of a metal ladle, hit the nuts until they are coarsely broken up. Flip the bag over and smash again; do this a few more times until the pieces are to your preferred size.

Per Serving: Calories: 305; Total Fat: 15g; Saturated Fat: 3g; Cholesterol: 55mg; Sodium: 472mg; Total Carbohydrates: 18g; Fiber: 3g; Protein: 27g

"I was skeptical about the yogurt base for the coating, but it worked quite well. I loved the flavor and crunch of the final dish!"

—Janice from Melrose, MA

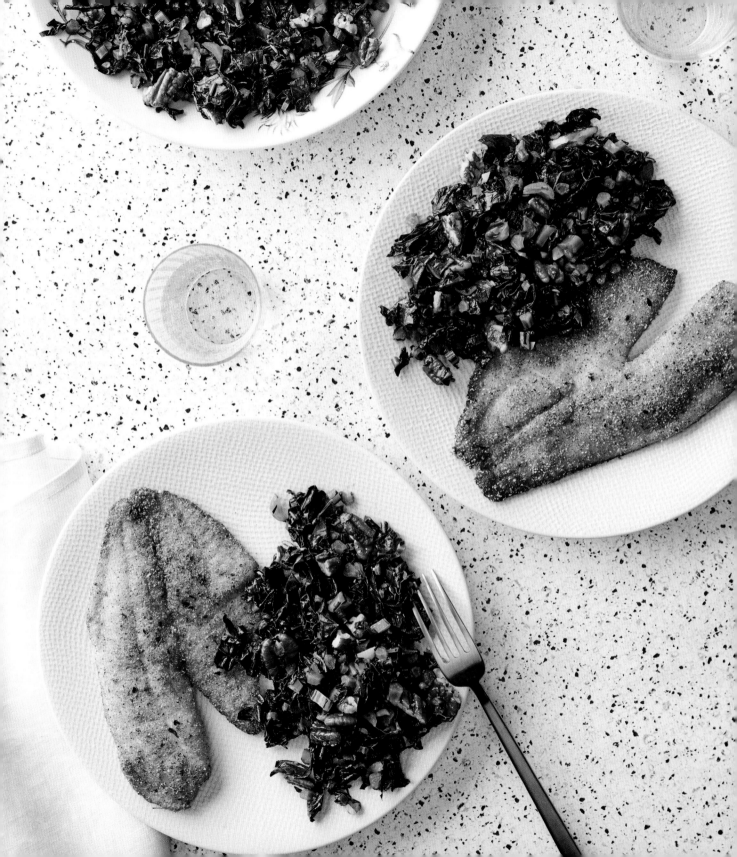

Blackened Tilapia with Honey-Pecan Greens

Dairy-Free, Gluten-Free, Egg-Free	Serves 4	Prep time: 15 minutes	Cook time: 25 minutes

1 bunch greens (such as collards, kale, Swiss chard, or mustard greens)

3 tablespoons extra-virgin olive oil, divided

2 garlic cloves, minced

¼ teaspoon crushed red pepper, divided

1 tablespoon honey

2 tablespoons cornmeal

½ teaspoon ground cumin

½ teaspoon dried oregano leaves

½ teaspoon smoked paprika

¼ teaspoon kosher or sea salt

¼ teaspoon black pepper

4 (4-ounce) tilapia fillets

½ cup Honey-Roasted Pecans with Thyme (page 41), chopped

Deanna calls this the double-whammy recipe—one that could turn around anyone who doesn't think they like fish or turns his or her nose up at dark leafy greens. Tilapia is a mild white fish that takes on the flavor of anything—in this case, a tantalizing mix of dried herbs and spices with the slight crunch of a cornmeal crust. And here those tough, hearty greens are mellowed out by a hit of honey and mixed with our irresistible Honey-Roasted Pecans with Thyme.

Lay 3 or 4 leaves of the greens on top of each other and fold in half so the stem is at the fold. Run your knife down the inside of the thick stems, removing them from the leaves. Repeat with the remaining leaves. Chop the stems into small slices. Set aside. Chop the leaves into ½-inch slices, keeping them separate from the sliced stems.

In a large stockpot over medium heat, heat 2 tablespoons of the olive oil. Add the sliced stems and cook, stirring occasionally, for 3 minutes. Add the garlic and ⅛ teaspoon of the crushed red pepper. Cook, stirring frequently, for 30 seconds. Add the chopped greens and honey, then stir well to coat. Cover and cook, stirring occasionally, until the greens completely soften, 15 minutes. Remove from the stove, uncover, and let cool in the pot for 5 to 10 minutes.

While the greens cook, in a cast iron skillet over medium-high heat, heat the remaining 1 tablespoon olive oil.

In a shallow bowl, mix together the cornmeal, cumin, oregano, smoked paprika, salt, black pepper, and remaining ⅛ teaspoon crushed red pepper. Dredge each piece of fish in the spice mixture until covered on each side. Carefully place into the hot skillet and cook for 3 minutes, then flip. Cook until the fish just starts to flake in the middle, 2 to 3 more minutes. Remove from the pan and place on a serving platter.

In a serving bowl, toss the cooked greens with the pecans and serve alongside the fish.

continued

Healthy Kitchen Hack: For a speedier version of the greens, use baby spinach, which doesn't have thick stems to remove. It cooks more quickly because it's a delicate green. That said, spinach cooks down quite a bit so we use double the amount (16 ounces) but with the same amount of olive oil, garlic, crushed red pepper, and honey. To cook, start by adding the garlic and crushed red pepper to the oil as directed. Once you add the spinach and honey, you'll only need 5 to 6 minutes of cooking time. After removing from the stove and allowing the spinach to cool down a bit, drain any liquid that may have accumulated at the bottom of the pot before mixing with the pecans.

Per Serving: Calories: 326; Total Fat: 21g; Saturated Fat: 3g; Cholesterol: 57mg; Sodium: 231mg; Total Carbohydrates: 14g; Fiber: 4g; Protein: 26g

Greek Seafood Rice Bowl

Nut-Free, Gluten-Free, Egg-Free | **Serves 4** | Prep time: 10 minutes | Cook time: 15 minutes

1 cup uncooked instant brown rice

2 tablespoons extra-virgin olive oil, divided

2 garlic cloves, minced

1 teaspoon dried oregano

1 pound frozen uncooked seafood medley (shrimp, calamari, scallops), thawed

¼ teaspoon kosher or sea salt

¼ teaspoon black pepper

1 medium lemon, cut in half

3 ounces feta cheese, crumbled

½ cup fresh mint leaves, chopped

1 large cucumber, chopped (about 2 cups)

Since Greece is the land of around 6,000 islands, it's not surprising that there are just about as many glorious Greek fish and shellfish recipes out there. For these bowls, we take advantage of a frozen seafood mix but if you can't find such a product, feel free to swap in frozen shrimp, scallops, mussels, or calamari. Be sure to thaw it ahead of time and look for the cooking time recommendation on the package to avoid overcooked, rubbery seafood.

Into a medium saucepan, measure the rice and 2¼ cups water. Bring to a boil over high heat, then reduce the heat to medium. Cover and cook until the water is absorbed, 10 to 12 minutes. Fluff the rice with a fork.

While the rice is cooking, place a large skillet over medium heat. Pour in 1 tablespoon of the oil and let it warm. Add the garlic and oregano and cook, stirring frequently, for 30 seconds. Add the seafood and cook until the shrimp just turns pink, 3 to 5 minutes (smaller shrimp will take less time to cook). Remove from the heat. Stir in the salt and black pepper.

Squeeze 1 tablespoon of the lemon juice into a large bowl. (Save any remaining lemon for another use.) Whisk in the remaining 1 tablespoon oil and add the cooked rice; stir well. Gently mix in the feta and mint.

To assemble, divide the rice among four bowls. Top with the cucumber and spoon the seafood and the pan liquid over the rice.

Healthy Kitchen Hack: Slash your cooking time in (more than!) half by swapping in couscous for the rice. (Bonus points if you can find whole-wheat couscous.) Bring ½ cup water to a boil in the saucepan then remove from the stove. Add ½ cup couscous and stir. Cover with a lid and let sit for 5 minutes. Fluff with a fork and mix in the lemon juice, olive oil, feta, and mint as instructed above.

Per Serving: Calories: 328; Total Fat: 13g; Saturated Fat: 4g; Cholesterol: 201mg; Sodium: 483mg; Total Carbohydrates: 27g; Fiber: 2g; Protein: 29g

Red Sea Shrimp with Salted Olive Oil Yogurt

| Nut-Free, Gluten-Free, Egg-Free | Serves 4 | Prep time: 10 minutes | Cook time: 5 minutes |

2 garlic cloves, minced

1 tablespoon honey

2 teaspoons chili powder

1 teaspoon ground cumin

1 teaspoon smoked paprika

¼ teaspoon black pepper

1 pound frozen uncooked large shrimp, thawed, peeled, and tails removed

4 tablespoons extra-virgin olive oil, divided

2 cups plain 2% Greek yogurt (16 ounces)

½ teaspoon kosher or sea salt

¼ cup chopped fresh cilantro

1 medium lemon, cut in half

While the Red Sea is clearly not the Mediterranean Sea, these bodies of water are only a few hundred kilometers apart. This shrimp dish was inspired by an incredible Israeli fish restaurant that Deanna and her travel companion stumbled upon in the port city of Eilat at the tip of the Red Sea. The ambiance was magical with a view of the vibrant blue water; and the seafood was a revelation—like this idea of pairing spicy shellfish with smooth, creamy yogurt. This is one of Deanna's very favorite recipes in the entire book!

In a large bowl, mix together the garlic, honey, chili powder, cumin, smoked paprika, and black pepper. Add the shrimp and toss well to coat.

In a large skillet over medium heat, heat 1 tablespoon of the olive oil. Add the shrimp and cook, stirring occasionally, until the shrimp just turn pink, 5 to 6 minutes. Remove from the heat.

While the shrimp cook, in a small bowl, add the yogurt, 6 tablespoons water, and the salt. Whisk together and then divide evenly among four shallow serving bowls. Drizzle the yogurt with the remaining 3 tablespoons olive oil.

When the shrimp is ready, divide it equally among the four bowls, placing it in the middle of the yogurt. Sprinkle with the cilantro and give each bowl a squeeze of juice from one half of the lemon. (Save the other lemon half for another use.)

Healthy Kitchen Hack: To make a vegetarian version (Red Sea Chickpeas), swap in a 15-ounce can of chickpeas (drained and rinsed) for the shrimp. Toss with the same spices and then heat in the skillet with 1 tablespoon olive oil until warm, 2 to 3 minutes. Serve with the salted olive oil yogurt, cilantro, and lemon juice.

Per Serving: Calories: 324; Total Fat: 17g; Saturated Fat: 4g; Cholesterol: 194mg; Sodium: 453mg; Total Carbohydrates: 10g; Fiber: 1g; Protein: 35g

Oven-Baked Fish Piccata with Parmesan Polenta

Nut-Free, Gluten-Free, Egg-Free	Serves 4	Prep time: 10 minutes	Cook time: 15 minutes

1 (18-ounce) tube plain polenta

3 tablespoons extra-virgin olive oil, divided

1½ tablespoons grated Parmesan or Pecorino Romano cheese

1 medium lemon, cut in half

2 tablespoons dry white wine

1 pound white fish fillet (skin-on or skinless) such as cod, tilapia, grouper, or snapper, cut into 4 total pieces

2 tablespoons capers from a jar, drained and rinsed

¼ teaspoon kosher or sea salt

¼ teaspoon black pepper

While you'll need two baking sheets to make this recipe, the entire meal is cooked in the oven so there'll be no extra skillets or saucepans to wash. Piccata sauce is traditionally made on the stovetop with lemon juice, capers, and butter, but here we bake it in the oven and swap in olive oil for the butter. We serve it next to sliced polenta with an irresistible baked cheese crust, which is an easy-to-make whole-grain side dish for any meat, chicken, fish, or plant protein.

Preheat the oven to 400°F. Line two large rimmed baking sheets with aluminum foil. Coat both with cooking spray.

Cut the polenta tube into 16 even slices. Arrange the slices in a single layer on one of the prepared baking sheets. Brush the tops with 1 tablespoon of the olive oil and sprinkle them with the Parmesan cheese. Set aside.

Squeeze 2 tablespoons of lemon juice into a large bowl. (Save any remaining lemon for another use.) Add the remaining 2 tablespoons olive oil and the wine and mix together. With tongs, add the fish pieces and turn a few times to evenly coat. Place the fish pieces skin-side down (if there is skin) on the other prepared baking sheet and drizzle the liquid from the bowl on top. Sprinkle with the capers, salt, and black pepper.

Put the fish and the polenta in the oven on separate oven racks. Bake for 10 to 12 minutes for thinner fish like tilapia, 12 to 14 minutes for thicker fish like cod, or until the pieces just barely start to flake in the thickest part. Bake the polenta for 10 to 15 minutes.

To serve, place four polenta slices on one side of each of four plates. Place a piece of fish next to the polenta on each plate. Drizzle the fish with any remaining sauce from the pan.

Healthy Kitchen Hack: As they do in the Mediterranean, we use *a lot* of fresh lemons in this book. We strongly recommend using superior-tasting fresh

continued

lemons over bottled lemon juice. And to reduce food waste, save any extra lemon juice or zest for the next recipe! Get in the habit of always grating lemon zest before juicing lemons, even when the recipe doesn't call for the zest. Simply stash extra zest for up to 6 months in the freezer in a freezer-proof container. Lemon juice will keep in the refrigerator for about 2 weeks or in the freezer for up to 3 months. (Freeze in ice cube trays!)

Per Serving: Calories: 291; Total Fat: 13g; Saturated Fat: 3g; Cholesterol: 58mg; Sodium: 576mg; Total Carbohydrates: 19g; Fiber: 4g; Protein: 25g

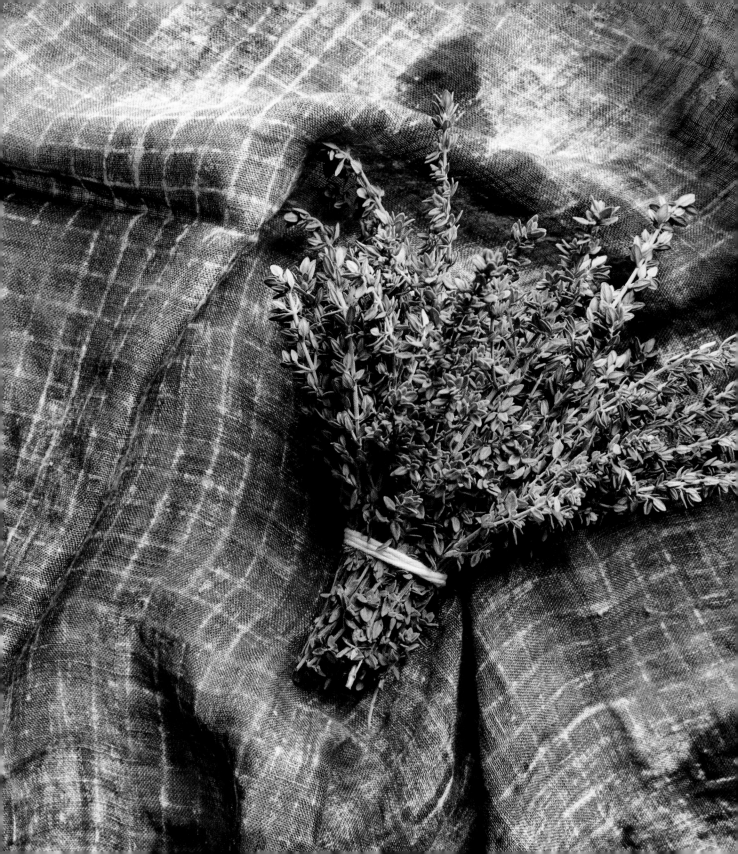

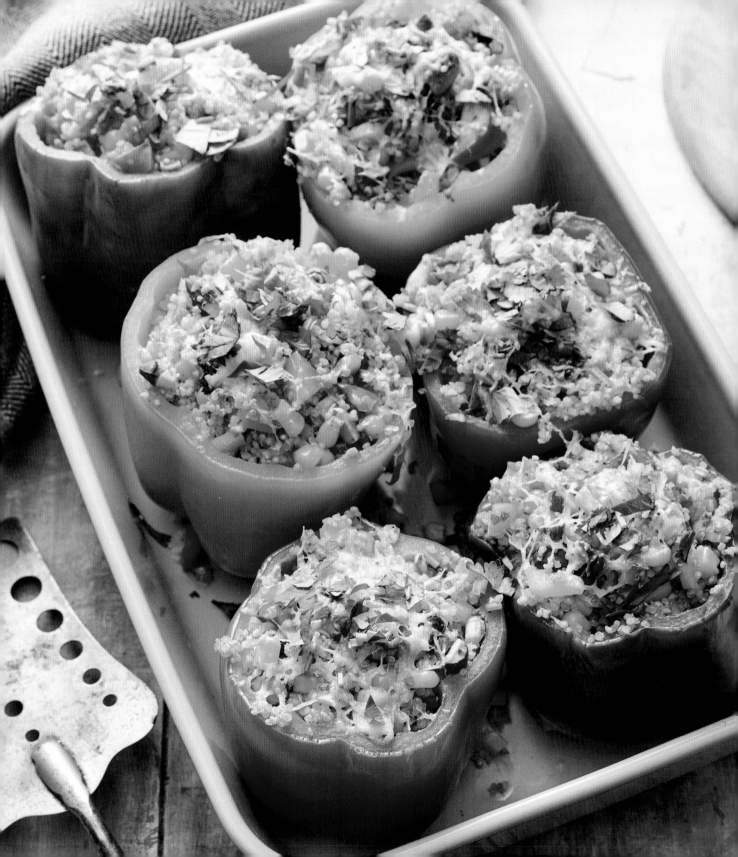

vegetable mains

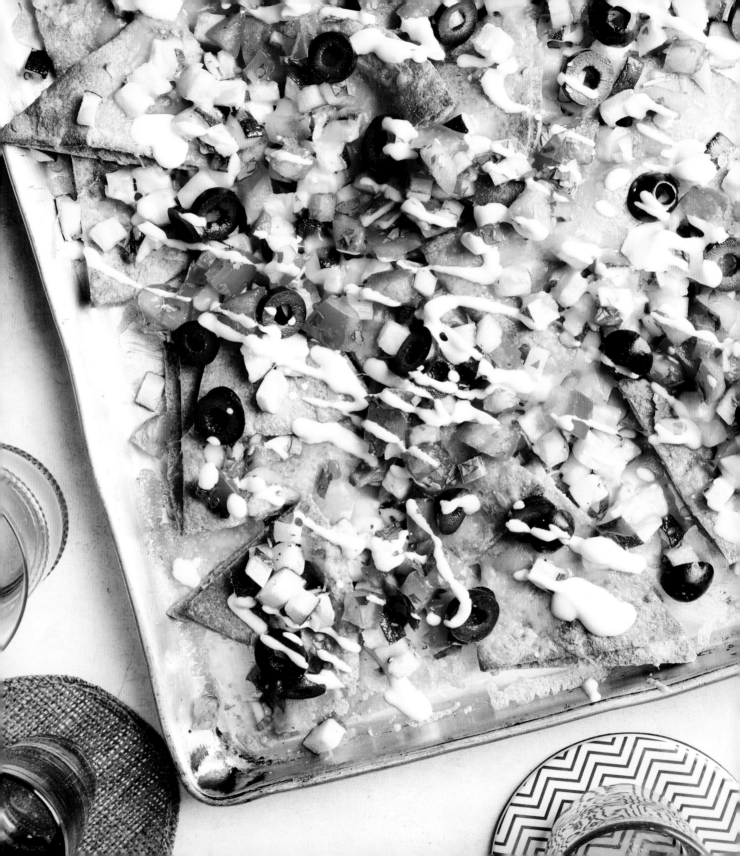

Greek Zucchini Pita Nachos

Nut-Free, Egg-Free, Vegetarian | Serves 4 | Prep time: 10 minutes | Cook time: 20 minutes

3 cups diced zucchini (about 2 medium zucchini)

2 garlic cloves, minced

1 tablespoon extra-virgin olive oil

¼ teaspoon kosher or sea salt

¼ teaspoon black pepper

4 whole-wheat pita rounds, each cut into 6 wedges

1 cup chopped tomato

¼ cup diced red onion

2 tablespoons chopped fresh cilantro

¾ cup plain 2% Greek yogurt (about 6 ounces)

1 (2.25-ounce) can sliced black olives (about ½ cup), 2 tablespoons of the liquid from the can reserved

1 cup shredded cheese like Monterey Jack, Colby Jack, or cheddar (about 4 ounces)

We often combine different cuisines together in our kitchens, and here Tex-Mex meets Mediterranean because we love nachos that much. Use up your summer zucchini in this better-for-you-snack-turned-into-a-meal recipe with a Greek twist.

Preheat the oven to 400°F. Coat a large rimmed baking sheet with cooking spray.

In a large bowl, toss the zucchini, garlic, olive oil, salt, and black pepper to combine. Spread onto the prepared baking pan. Roast for 10 minutes, stirring halfway through.

While the zucchini is cooking, place the pita wedges on a wire rack. Set the rack on another baking sheet and then put it into the oven right after stirring the zucchini. Bake the pita wedges for 5 minutes.

While the zucchini and pita bake, mix together the tomato, onion, and cilantro in a bowl; set the salsa aside. In another bowl, whisk together the yogurt and the olive can liquid.

Remove the zucchini and pita from the oven. Turn on the broiler to high.

Remove the rack with the pita wedges from the baking sheet, then carefully arrange the pita wedges on the now empty hot pan. Spoon the roasted zucchini over the pita wedges and top with the cheese. Broil, watching closely so as not to burn the pita, for 1½ to 2 minutes, until the cheese is melted. Remove from the broiler.

To assemble, spoon the salsa over the melted cheese. Then spoon the yogurt sauce over the salsa. Top the nachos with the olives and serve.

continued

Greek Zucchini Pita Nachos (continued)

Healthy Kitchen Hack: Plain Greek yogurt is a more nutritious option compared to sour cream, but still delivers that cool and creamy mouthfeel.

Per Serving: Calories: 380; Total Fat: 17g; Saturated Fat: 7g; Cholesterol: 32mg; Sodium: 1,021mg; Total Carbohydrates: 44g; Fiber: 5g; Protein: 18g

"Usually I don't cook much, but this recipe was actually fun to assemble, and I was able to add in the vegetables my family likes. My husband skipped the yogurt topping but everyone else enjoyed it!"

—Eileen from La Grange Park, IL

Mushroom, Leek, and Walnut Israeli Couscous

Egg-Free, Vegetarian		Serves 4	Prep time: 5 minutes	Cook time: 25 minutes

2 tablespoons extra-virgin olive oil, divided

1 (8-ounce) box whole-wheat or regular Israeli couscous (about 1⅓ cups)

2 cups low-sodium or no-salt-added vegetable broth, divided

2 cups chopped white button or baby bella mushrooms

2 large leeks

¼ teaspoon kosher or sea salt

¼ teaspoon black pepper

½ cup walnut pieces

¼ cup grated Parmesan cheese (about 1 ounce)

Leeks are related to onions but are much milder, and they take on a lovely buttery flavor when cooked into recipes like this simple yet satisfying grain dish. Rinse them well as leeks are grown in a sandy dirt and the grit can get trapped in their layers. If you don't have leeks on hand, you can swap in sweet onions, like Vidalia or Walla Walla.

In a medium saucepan, heat 1 tablespoon of the olive oil over medium heat. Add the couscous and stir until lightly browned.

Add 1¾ cups of the broth. Bring to a boil, then cover the pan with a lid and reduce the heat to low. Cook for 12 minutes, then remove the pan from the heat and fluff the couscous with a fork.

While the couscous is cooking, heat the remaining 1 tablespoon olive oil in a large skillet over medium heat. Add the mushrooms and cook, stirring occasionally, for 5 minutes.

While the mushrooms cook, slice each leek in half lengthwise and rinse well in water to remove all the dirt. Thinly slice the white and light green parts and discard the tough dark green parts. (See page 19 for ideas on using food scraps.)

Add the leeks, salt, and pepper to the skillet with the mushrooms and cook, stirring occasionally, until the leeks have softened, 7 to 8 minutes.

While the leeks and mushrooms cook, put the walnuts in a small skillet over medium heat. Cook, stirring occasionally, until the walnuts are lightly toasted, 4 to 6 minutes. Set aside.

Pour the remaining ¼ cup broth into the leek-mushroom mixture and cook, stirring occasionally, until it reduces in volume, 2 to 3 minutes. Remove from the heat and add to a large serving bowl. Pour in the couscous and mix together gently. Mix in the toasted walnuts and the cheese and serve.

continued

Healthy Kitchen Hack: Similar to toasting nuts, toasting grains adds another layer of flavor to your dishes. You can toast grains like oats, quinoa, bulgur, farro, rice, and barley in a little olive oil or in a dry pan over medium heat. Toast, stirring frequently to prevent burning, for 2 to 5 minutes or until the grains smell nutty. Then cook the grains according to your recipe. Try toasting the barley for the Lemon Barley Pilaf on page 213 or the quinoa for the Spanish-Style Stuffed Peppers on page 209.

Per Serving: Calories: 406; Total Fat: 19g; Saturated Fat: 3g; Cholesterol: 4mg; Sodium: 282mg; Total Carbohydrates: 49g; Fiber: 5g; Protein: 13g

"I made this while visiting my sister, and we both *loved* it! The mushrooms added a wonderful meaty flavor. I also substituted acini de pepe pasta for the couscous and it still turned out great."

—Donna from Havertown, PA

Tuscan Beans over Polenta

Nut-Free, Gluten-Free, Egg-Free, Vegetarian	Serves 6	Prep time: 10 minutes	Cook time: 10 minutes

2 (15-ounce) cans cannellini or great northern beans, drained, liquid reserved

1 tablespoon extra-virgin olive oil

2 garlic cloves, minced

6 fresh sage leaves, finely chopped (about 1½ tablespoons)

⅛ teaspoon crushed red pepper

¼ teaspoon kosher or sea salt

¼ teaspoon black pepper

2 (18-ounce) tubes plain polenta

¼ cup grated Parmesan or Pecorino Romano cheese (about 1 ounce)

While it's not the prettiest dish, this hearty vegetarian meal entices with the alluring flavors of Tuscany. If you can't find sage, chopped fresh rosemary would be just as lovely. Serve it with our Tomato-Onion Plate with Mint (page 87) and enjoy with a glass of Chianti—*buon appetito*!

In a colander, rinse the beans well in the sink under cold water. Set aside.

Heat the olive oil in a medium saucepan over medium heat. Add the garlic, sage, and crushed red pepper and cook, stirring constantly, for 30 seconds. Add the beans, salt, black pepper, and ¼ cup of the reserved bean liquid. Stir well, reduce the heat to medium-low, and keep warm until the polenta is ready.

While the beans cook, remove the polenta from the plastic wrapping. Slice one tube of the polenta into ½-inch-thick rounds and place in a microwave-safe bowl. Microwave on high for 45 seconds. Transfer the polenta to a large stockpot and repeat with the second tube of polenta, then add that to the pot as well and mash with a potato masher or fork until coarsely mashed. Place the pot over medium heat.

Pour the remaining bean liquid into a liquid measuring cup and add enough water to make 1 cup of liquid. Whisk the liquid into the polenta until completely absorbed. Heat the polenta until warm, 2 to 3 minutes. Remove from the heat and stir the cheese into the polenta until melted.

To serve, spoon the polenta into bowls and top with the Tuscan beans.

Healthy Kitchen Hack: Adapt this recipe into a quick Tuscan bean soup! Cook the beans as above, then heat with 6 to 8 cups of low sodium broth, depending on desired soup consistency. When hot, add 3 cups chopped kale or spinach and simmer for 10 minutes. Serve with grated cheese.

Per Serving: Calories: 274; Total Fat: 4g; Saturated Fat: 1g; Cholesterol: 4mg; Sodium: 824mg; Total Carbohydrates: 49g; Fiber: 9g; Protein: 10g

Broccoli-Cheese Risotto

| Nut-Free, Egg-Free, Vegetarian | Serves 6 | Prep time: 5 minutes | Cook time: 20 minutes |

3½ cups low-sodium or no-salt-added vegetable broth

1 tablespoon extra-virgin olive oil

4 garlic cloves, minced

2 cups uncooked quick-cooking or instant pearl barley

½ cup dry white wine or broth (see Healthy Kitchen Hack below)

1 (16-ounce) package frozen broccoli

1¼ cups grated Parmesan or Pecorino Romano cheese (about 5 ounces), divided

¼ teaspoon kosher or sea salt

¼ teaspoon black pepper

Chopped fresh chives and lemon wedges, for serving (optional)

Barley is a great stand-in for Italian risotto rice as it turns into a similar bowl of comfort food when cooked. We always have frozen produce on hand for last-minute dinners like this recipe. Frozen vegetables cut down on food waste because they are already trimmed and plus, they won't rot away forgotten in the refrigerator. Most frozen veggies can be added straight to your pot of cooked grains, no thawing necessary, which helps them retain their natural color, too.

Pour the broth into a medium saucepan and bring to a simmer over low heat.

In a large stockpot over medium-high heat, heat the olive oil. Add the garlic and cook, stirring occasionally, for 1 minute. Add the barley and cook, stirring occasionally, until the barley begins to toast, about 2 minutes. Pour in the wine and cook until most of the liquid evaporates.

Add 1 cup of the warm broth from the saucepan to the stockpot and cook, stirring frequently, until most of the liquid is absorbed, about 3 minutes. Add the remaining warm broth, turn the heat to high, and bring to a boil. Reduce the heat to medium-low, cover, and cook the barley for 6 minutes. Add the frozen broccoli and stir. Cook until the barley and broccoli have just softened, 4 to 6 more minutes. (For softer barley and broccoli, cook for an additional 5 to 10 minutes. Note: The broccoli will turn olive-green in color if cooked longer.)

Remove the pot from the heat and stir in 1 cup of the cheese, the salt, and the black pepper. Serve with the remaining cheese on the side, along with chives and lemon wedges, if desired.

continued

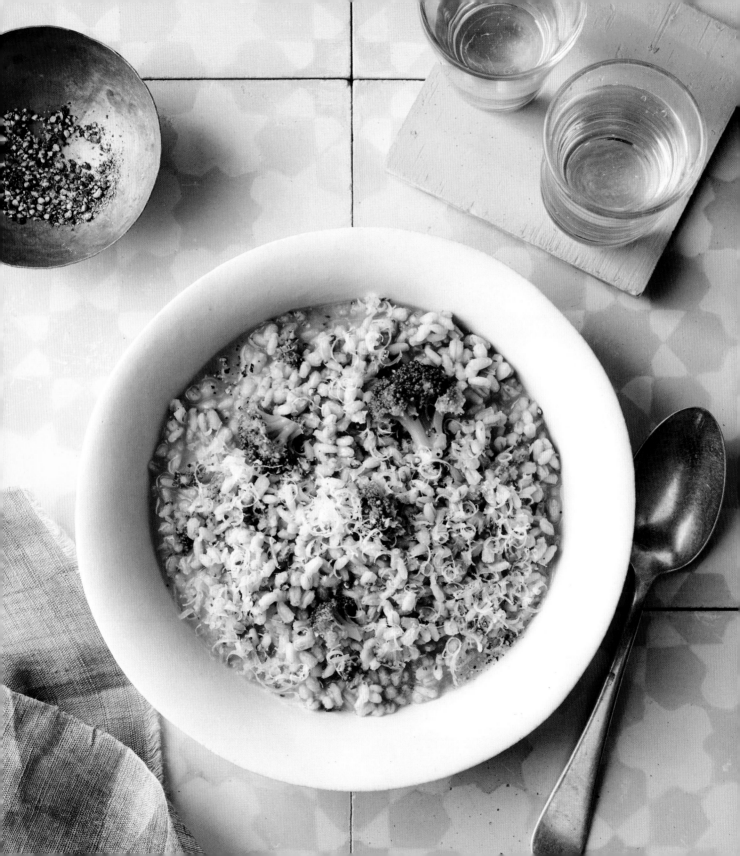

Broccoli-Cheese Risotto (continued)

Healthy Kitchen Hack: If you don't have an open bottle of white wine on hand, try these substitutions: for every ½ cup white wine, use ½ cup vegetable broth, ½ cup water with ½ teaspoon grated lemon zest, or ½ cup water with 1 tablespoon lemon juice.

Per Serving: Calories: 319; Total Fat: 10g; Saturated Fat: 4g; Cholesterol: 25mg; Total Carbohydrates: 45g; Fiber 8g; Protein 15g

"How could something this simple be so good? I like that it has some green veggies (something I should be eating more). Another bonus with this recipe: no onions to chop!"

–Zach from Charlotte, NC

Zucchini-Chickpea Couscous with Pistachio-Yogurt Sauce

Egg-Free, Vegetarian	Serves 4	Prep time: 5 minutes	Cook time: 15 minutes

2 tablespoons extra-virgin olive oil

1 garlic clove, minced

2 large zucchini, cut into ¼-inch pieces

1½ cups low-sodium vegetable broth, divided

1 (15-ounce) can chickpeas, drained and rinsed

½ teaspoon black pepper

¼ teaspoon kosher or sea salt

1 cup uncooked regular or whole-wheat couscous

¼ cup finely chopped dried apricots

1 medium lemon, cut in half

½ cup shelled pistachios

½ cup fresh mint leaves, divided

3 tablespoons plain 2% Greek yogurt

This dish has a surprising ingredient: dried apricots. While it might seem unusual to pair a sweet ingredient with zucchini and beans, Middle Eastern dishes often combine fruit like apricots, figs, raisins, or dates with grains, vegetables, meat, or poultry. To keep this vegetarian, we've added chickpeas as the main protein source, but you could swap in chicken or pork if you'd like.

In a large skillet over medium heat, heat the olive oil for 1 minute. Add the garlic and cook, stirring frequently, for 30 seconds. Add in the zucchini and cook, stirring occasionally, until the zucchini starts to soften, about 5 minutes. Pour in ¼ cup of the broth and the chickpeas; stir and cook for 5 more minutes. Remove the skillet from the heat and mix in the black pepper and salt.

While the zucchini cooks, make the couscous. In a medium saucepan, bring the remaining 1¼ cups of the broth to a boil. Pour in the couscous, remove the pot from the heat, and cover. Let it sit for 5 minutes, then stir with a fork. Mix in the dried apricots.

To make the pistachio-yogurt sauce, squeeze the juice from one lemon half into a high-powered blender or food processor. Add the pistachios, ¼ cup of the mint, the yogurt, and ¼ cup water. Process until smooth. If you like your sauce thinner, add 1 to 2 tablespoons more water.

To serve, spoon the couscous into four individual bowls. Top with the zucchini-chickpea mixture and drizzle with the pistachio-yogurt sauce. Tear up the remaining ¼ cup mint and sprinkle over each bowl. Cut the remaining lemon half into four wedges and serve one wedge with each bowl.

continued

Zucchini-Chickpea Couscous with Pistachio-Yogurt Sauce (continued)

Healthy Kitchen Hack: Expand your yogurt horizons! Think of Greek yogurt as a savory condiment, like in this recipe, instead of just a sweet breakfast ingredient. Mix it with your favorite herbs and spices then rub it on chicken as a marinade or swap it in for mayo on sandwiches. Check out our Olive Oil–Yogurt Spread on page (42) for even more unique savory uses.

Per Serving: Calories: 453; Total Fat: 16g; Saturated Fat: 2g; Cholesterol: 1mg; Sodium: 417mg; Total Carbohydrates: 63g; Fiber: 10g; Protein: 16g

"My husband and I really enjoyed this vegetarian dish! We especially liked the sauce, which brought all the elements of the recipe together."

—Alice from Lincoln, NE

Spiced Carrot Hummus Bowls

Egg-Free, Vegetarian		Serves 6	Prep time 15 minutes	Cook time: 25 minutes

1 cup uncooked farro

½ teaspoon kosher or sea salt, divided

4 medium carrots

2 tablespoons extra-virgin olive oil, divided

½ teaspoon ground cumin

½ teaspoon ground cinnamon

½ teaspoon smoked paprika, divided

¼ teaspoon black pepper

½ cup plain 2% Greek yogurt (4 ounces)

1 (10-ounce) container hummus or homemade hummus (see Healthy Kitchen Hack on page 50)

⅓ cup chopped almonds

⅓ cup fresh mint leaves, torn

Get out of your carrot-stick rut with this hearty, healthy, and craveable grain bowl. Roasting these carrots with a Mediterranean spice combo of cumin, cinnamon, and smoked paprika may have you eating them straight off the pan even before they get paired with the chewy farro, crunchy almonds, and fresh mint. We recommended you make an extra batch for munching and also to whip up the super-easy carrot soup featured in our Healthy Kitchen Hack below.

Place a large rimmed baking sheet on the middle rack in the oven. Preheat the oven to 450°F.

Into a medium saucepan, measure 2 cups water, the farro, and ¼ teaspoon of the salt. Bring to a boil over high heat. Reduce the heat to medium-low, cover, and cook until the farro is tender and chewy, 20 to 25 minutes.

While the farro cooks, cut the carrots into ¾-inch-thick slices, halving any slices that are larger than about ¾ inch in diameter. In a large bowl, mix together 1 tablespoon of the olive oil, the cumin, cinnamon, ¼ teaspoon of the smoked paprika, ⅛ teaspoon of the salt, and the black pepper. Add the carrots and mix well until coated.

Carefully remove the baking sheet from the oven and coat with cooking spray. Spread the carrots over the pan and roast for 10 minutes, stirring halfway through.

While the carrots cook, in a medium bowl, mix the yogurt, remaining 1 tablespoon olive oil, and remaining ⅛ teaspoon salt. Set aside.

In a small bowl, mix the hummus and remaining ¼ teaspoon smoked paprika.

To assemble, spoon the cooked farro into four bowls. Placing each in separate sections over each farro bowl, add the roasted carrots, yogurt spread, hummus, and almonds. Top with the mint and serve.

continued

Spiced Carrot Hummus Bowls (continued)

Healthy Kitchen Hack: Roasted carrot soup is a favorite soup at the Ball house. To make it, double the amount of carrots in this recipe, but keep the same amount of spices. After roasting, puree the carrots in a blender or food processor along with a 15-ounce can of beans (any kind, drained), 2 cups low-sodium vegetable broth, and 1 cup water. Warm the soup in the microwave or on the stovetop.

Per Serving: Calories: 471; Total Fat: 21g; Saturated Fat: 3g; Cholesterol: 3mg; Sodium: 461mg; Total Carbohydrates: 59g; Fiber: 11g; Protein: 17g

Spanish-Style Stuffed Peppers

Gluten-Free, Egg-Free, Vegetarian	Serves 6	Prep time: 10 minutes	Cook time: 25 minutes

1 cup uncooked quinoa

2 cups low-sodium or no-salt-added vegetable broth

¼ teaspoon kosher or sea salt

6 large bell peppers, any color

1 (15-ounce) can corn kernels, drained and rinsed

¾ cup grated Manchego cheese (about 3 ounces), divided

½ cup dry-roasted almonds, chopped

½ teaspoon smoked paprika

½ cup chopped fresh cilantro, divided

Okay, we realize quinoa is not from Spain, but this South American plant (which is actually a seed but because of its nutrient properties is consider a pseudo-whole grain) can still certainly be a part of the Mediterranean style of eating. It's especially good in vegetarian dishes, as it's packed with protein. We round out this recipe with Spanish staples like almonds, peppers, and smoked paprika (Deanna's favorite spice) to bring to mind the sunny Mediterranean—or sunny South America: your choice!

In a fine-mesh strainer, rinse the quinoa under running water to remove its natural bitter coating.

In a large stockpot, add the quinoa, broth, and salt. Bring to a boil, then reduce the heat, cover, and simmer until the broth is almost completely absorbed, 12 to 15 minutes. Remove from the heat.

While the quinoa is cooking, preheat the oven to 450°F.

Slice off the top of each bell pepper and cut the extra flesh from around the stem. Discard the stems. Finely chop the extra flesh and set aside for the stuffing. Remove the seeds from the inside of each pepper.

Place the peppers in a 9-inch square glass baking dish or round pie plate. Cover the dish with plastic wrap and poke a few holes in the wrap for ventilation. Microwave on high for 5 to 6 minutes, until the peppers are tender. Using oven mitts, remove the hot dish from the microwave and set on a wire rack.

When the quinoa is ready, mix in the reserved chopped bell pepper, corn, ½ cup of the cheese, the almonds, smoked paprika, and ¼ cup of the cilantro. Stuff the mixture into the cavity of each pepper. Carefully place the peppers standing up in the same baking dish (using an oven mitt to hold the dish if it's still too warm to touch). Sprinkle with the remaining cheese.

continued

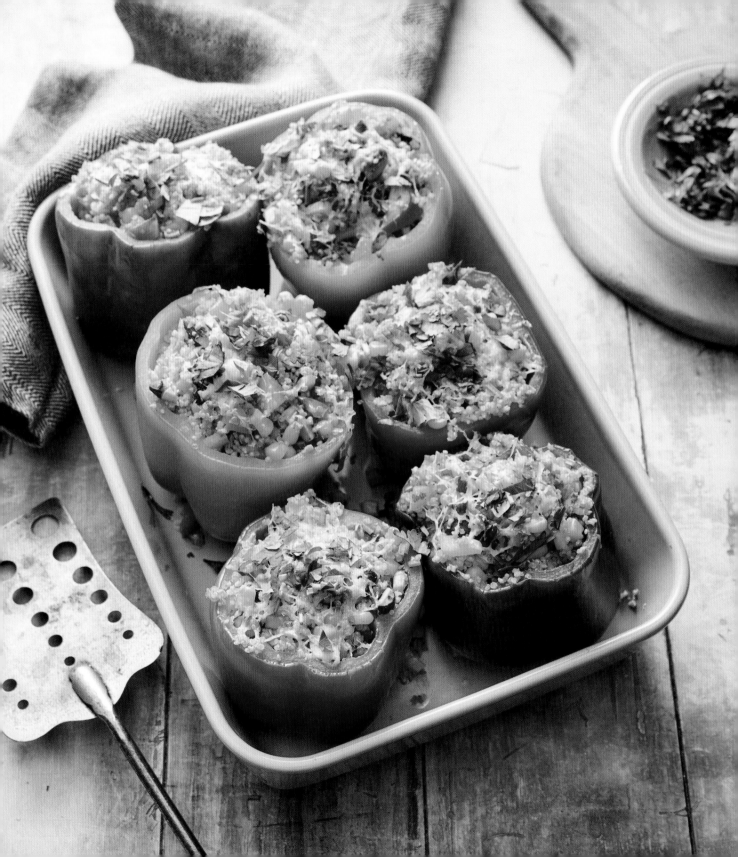

Bake for 10 minutes, until the peppers begin to look roasted and the cheese on top is melted. Sprinkle with the remaining ¼ cup cilantro before serving.

Healthy Kitchen Hack: Using the microwave to kick-start cooking your stuffed peppers eliminates at least 15 minutes of oven time. Try this method when making stuffed tomatoes, stuffed zucchini, or stuffed eggplant (knowing that the cooking times will vary depending on the size and firmness of each vegetable).

Per Serving: Calories: 343; Total Fat: 13g; Saturated Fat: 3g; Cholesterol: 11mg; Sodium: 385mg; Total Carbohydrates: 47g; Fiber: 9g; Protein: 14g

Weekday Eggplant Parmesan

Nut-Free, Gluten-Free, Egg-Free, Vegetarian	Serves 4	Prep time: 10 minutes	Cook time: 20 minutes

1 large globe eggplant (about 1 pound), stem sliced off

1½ tablespoons extra-virgin olive oil

½ teaspoon black pepper, divided

¼ teaspoon kosher or sea salt

1 (14.5-ounce) can low-sodium or no-salt-added crushed tomatoes with basil

1 (14.5-ounce) can low-sodium or no-salt-added diced tomatoes

2 teaspoons dried oregano

¾ cup shredded mozzarella cheese (about 3 ounces)

3 tablespoons grated Parmesan or Pecorino Romano cheese

¼ cup chopped fresh basil leaves (8 to 10 leaves)

When Deanna got her first apartment out of college, eggplant Parmesan was one of the go-to dinners in her weekly recipe rotation. Fast-forward to many years later: She's updated this dish to utilize the broiler to cut the cooking time in half.

Place the top oven rack about 4 inches below the broiler. Preheat the broiler to high. Coat a large rimmed baking sheet with cooking spray.

Slice the eggplant in half lengthwise. Slice each half into ¼-inch-thick half-moons and place them on the prepared baking sheet. Brush with half of the olive oil; sprinkle with ¼ teaspoon of the black pepper and the salt.

Broil the eggplant for 4 minutes. Using tongs, flip each slice and then brush with the remaining olive oil. Broil for 4 to 5 minutes, until golden brown. Remove the baking sheet from the oven and reduce the oven temperature to 450°F.

While the eggplant is cooking, put the crushed tomatoes, diced tomatoes, oregano, and remaining black pepper into a medium saucepan and mix well. Bring the sauce to a simmer over medium heat, stirring occasionally.

To assemble, cover the bottom of a 9-inch square baking pan with half the tomato sauce. Place the eggplant over the top, slightly overlapping each slice. Cover with the remaining sauce. Sprinkle with the mozzarella and then the Parmesan. Bake for 10 minutes, until bubbly. Remove from the oven and cool slightly. Sprinkle with the basil and serve.

Healthy Kitchen Hack: In the summer we like to swap in zucchini, summer squash, and tomato slices for some of the eggplant. Under the broiler, thin-skinned squash has a shorter cooking time than eggplant, 5 to 6 minutes total, and tomatoes only need 3 to 4 minutes total.

Per Serving: Calories: 270; Total Fat: 12g; Saturated Fat: 5g; Cholesterol: 22mg; Sodium: 668mg; Total Carbohydrates: 29g; Fiber: 8g; Protein: 14g

Lemon-Barley Pilaf with Grilled Portobello Mushrooms

Dairy-Free, Nut-Free, Egg-Free, Vegan | Serves 6 | Prep time: 5 minutes | Cook time: 25 minutes

2 tablespoons extra-virgin olive oil, divided

1 cup diced onion (about ½ medium onion)

2 cups chopped baby bella mushrooms (about 8 ounces)

2 cups uncooked quick-cooking or instant pearl barley

½ teaspoon kosher or sea salt

¼ teaspoon black pepper

3 sprigs thyme (about 1 tablespoon fresh thyme leaves) or 1 teaspoon dried thyme

1 medium lemon, cut in half

6 portobello mushrooms, stems and gills removed

We think this recipe will make you and your family fans of barley if you aren't eating it already! It's got a nutty, hearty flavor and one serving of barley provides a notable amount of protein and fiber. It can also be swapped for rice (with adjusted cooking times). We serve this pilaf with meaty portobello mushrooms, though Serena's husband also loves it as a side dish with a small steak.

In a large stockpot over medium-high heat, heat 1 tablespoon of the olive oil. Add the onion and cook, stirring occasionally, for 5 minutes. Add the chopped mushrooms and cook, stirring occasionally, until some of the liquid they release evaporates, 4 to 5 minutes.

Stir in 4 cups water, the barley, salt, pepper, and thyme sprigs, increase the heat to high, and bring to a boil. Cover with a lid, reduce the heat to medium-low, and cook for 8 minutes. Keep the pot covered and remove from the heat; let the pot sit until all the liquid is absorbed and the barley is tender, 4 to 5 minutes. Squeeze 1 tablespoon of lemon juice into the pot and stir well. (Save any remaining lemon for another use.) Using tongs, carefully remove the thyme sprigs and strip off any remaining leaves into the pot.

While the barley is cooking, heat a grill to medium-high or heat a grill pan over medium-high heat. Brush the remaining olive oil over both sides of the portobello mushroom caps. Place the mushrooms bottom-side down (where the stem was removed) on the grill or pan. Cover and cook for 5 minutes. (If using a grill pan, grill in two batches using a sheet of aluminum foil as a cover.) Flip the mushroom caps over, cover, and grill until tender, 2 to 3 minutes.

Using a spatula, transfer the mushroom caps, bottom-side up, to individual serving plates. Fill each cap with the barley pilaf and serve.

continued

Lemon-Barley Pilaf with Grilled Portobello Mushrooms (continued)

Healthy Kitchen Hack: While fresh thyme is a savory herb that adds a ton of flavor, stripping off the leaves can be tedious. When using thyme in a cooked dish, throw in the entire stem with the leaves intact. Most of the leaves will fall off during the heating process and the few remaining leaves can be easily stripped off the stem after cooking and added to the dish.

Per Serving: Calories: 248; Total Fat: 6g; Saturated Fat: 1g; Cholesterol: 0mg; Sodium: 177 mg; Total Carbohydrates: 45g; Fiber: 7g; Protein: 8g

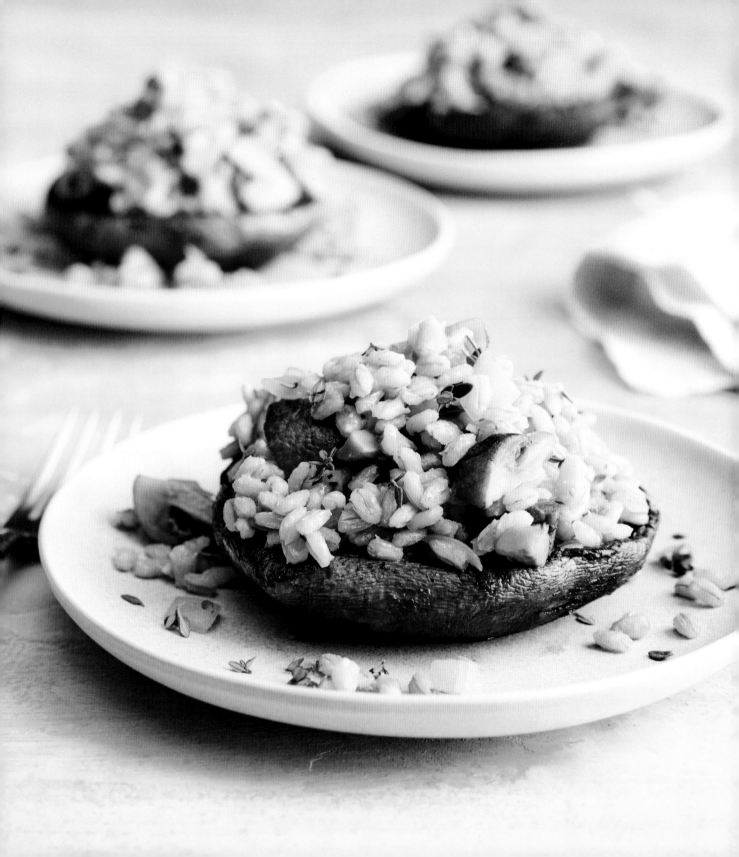

Sun-Dried Tomato Veggie Burgers

| Dairy-Free, Gluten-Free, Vegetarian | Serves 4 | Prep time: 10 minutes | Cook time: 20 minutes |

6 sun-dried tomatoes (dry from a pouch)

1 (15-ounce) can chickpeas, drained, liquid reserved

¼ cup gluten-free rolled oats (regular or quick-cooking)

1 large egg

1 tablespoon creamy peanut butter

1 tablespoon red wine vinegar

2 garlic cloves, minced

1 teaspoon ground cumin

¼ teaspoon kosher or sea salt, divided

¼ teaspoon black pepper

1 tablespoon extra-virgin olive oil

Peanut butter is the secret ingredient that gives these chickpea burgers a delicious nutty zip, and also helps bind them as they turn crispy and golden brown when cooking. We like to pair them with a cool bed of greens like our Herb Salad with Citrus-Date Dressing on page 73, for a lovely contrast of flavors and colors.

Place the sun-dried tomatoes in a small bowl and cover with ¼ cup boiling water; let them soften for at least 10 minutes. Remove from the water and finely chop.

Place the chopped tomatoes, chickpeas, 2 tablespoons of the reserved chickpea liquid, the oats, egg, peanut butter, vinegar, garlic, cumin, salt, and black pepper into a food processor. Process for 10 to 15 pulses until a sticky mixture forms. (Alternatively, in a large bowl, mash the chickpea mixture with a potato masher or fork until roughly smashed.)

Divide the mixture into 4 heaping ⅓-cup portions and place them onto a plate.

In a large nonstick skillet over medium-high heat, heat the olive oil until very hot, about 3 minutes. Gently slide the burger portions into the hot oil. Using a flat spatula, press each portion flat to about ¾ inch thick. Cook the patties for 4 minutes, then flip them with a spatula. Cook until golden brown, 3 to 4 minutes more. Serve over greens, if desired.

Healthy Kitchen Hack: For a different flavor slant, follow the above recipe using this formula: ¼ cup of your favorite chopped vegetable, 1 (15-ounce) can any type of beans, and different spices. For a Mexican veggie burger, use corn, pinto beans, and cumin. For an Italian version, use canned tomatoes (drained), cannellini beans, and oregano.

Per Serving: Calories: 300; Total Fat: 10g; Saturated Fat: 1g; Cholesterol: 47mg; Sodium: 606mg; Total Carbohydrates: 40g; Fiber: 11g; Protein: 14g

Spaghetti Squash Noodles with Chickpea "Meatballs"

Nut-Free, Egg-Free, Vegetarian	Serves 4	Prep time: 15 minutes	Cook time: 15 minutes

1 medium spaghetti squash

1 bunch (about 6) green onions

1 (15-ounce) can chickpeas, drained, liquid reserved

2 tablespoons chickpea flour or white whole-wheat flour

1 tablespoon dried oregano

¼ teaspoon kosher or sea salt

1 tablespoon extra-virgin olive oil

2 cups (16 ounces) jarred reduced-sodium pasta sauce or canned low-sodium pizza sauce

¼ cup grated Parmesan or Pecorino Romano cheese (about 1 ounce), for serving

Serena's children love spaghetti and meatballs, meaning pasta and meat, but this vegetarian version also gets two thumbs up from them. It's an easy and yummy way to get more veggies into your family's eating routine by way of spaghetti squash "noodles" and chickpea "meatballs" (which are actually more like mini patties than traditional round spheres).

Preheat the oven to 425°F. Place a large rimmed baking sheet in the oven to heat.

Using a small sharp knife, carefully poke a few holes in the squash and microwave on high for 5 minutes. Using oven mitts, remove the hot squash from the microwave and slice it in half lengthwise using a large sharp knife. Carefully remove the seeds (they will be hot).

Cover both squash halves with wet paper towels and place back in the microwave, cut-side up. Microwave on high for 7 to 10 minutes until the squash is barely tender.

Using oven mitts, remove the squash from the microwave and let cool for a few minutes. Scrape the flesh with a fork to separate it from the squash halves and create "noodles."

Roughly chop the green onions into 1-inch pieces. In a food processor, add the green onions, chickpeas, 1 tablespoon of the chickpea liquid, the flour, oregano, and salt. Pulse about 10 times until the mixture is combined (but not pureed); add more chickpea liquid if the mixture does not come together. Using a 1½-tablespoon scoop, spoon the mixture into 12 portions onto a plate.

Using oven mitts, remove the baking sheet from the oven and add the olive oil, tilting the pan from side to side to coat evenly with the oil. Using a fork, transfer the chickpea portions to the pan and gently flatten them with your fingers to make 2-inch patties. Bake the patties for 5 minutes; flip the patties and bake for 5 minutes more, until they start to turn golden brown.

continued

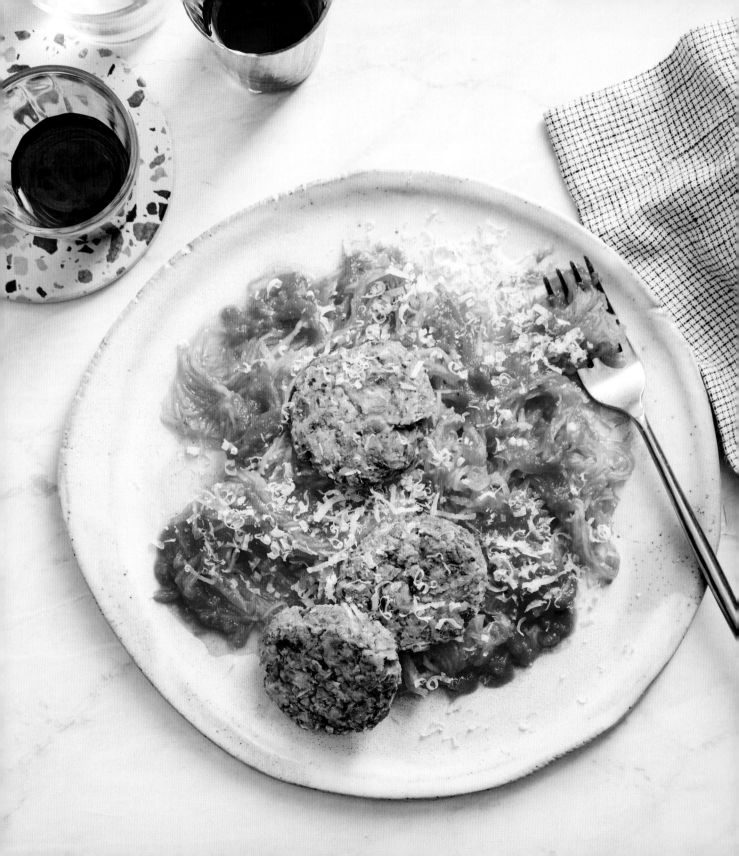

Spaghetti Squash Noodles with Chickpea "Meatballs" (continued)

While the chickpea patties are baking, place the spaghetti squash noodles and the pasta sauce in a large microwave-safe bowl and microwave for 3 to 5 minutes on 70 percent power, until warm. Serve the noodles and sauce with the chickpea "meatballs" and the cheese on the side.

Healthy Kitchen Hack: When cutting any type of winter squash, such as acorn, butternut, or spaghetti, use the microwave trick we feature to make it easier to slice through those tough skins. Cut a few small slits into the squash and then microwave it for about 5 minutes. Cut the squash in half lengthwise, then roast in the oven or continue microwaving until tender.

Per Serving: Calories: 388; Total Fat: 11g; Saturated Fat: 2g; Cholesterol: 4mg; Sodium: 1,052mg; Total Carbohydrates: 61g; Fiber: 16g; Protein: 16g

Artichoke-Cheese Strata

Nut-Free, Vegetarian	Serves 6	Prep time: 10 minutes	Cook time: 20 minutes

3 whole-wheat pita breads, cut into 1-inch square pieces

1 (14-ounce) can quartered artichoke hearts, drained

6 large eggs

1¼ cups reduced-fat (2%) milk

1 cup shredded Manchego or cheddar cheese (about 4 ounces)

2 tablespoons fresh dill or 2 teaspoons dried

¼ teaspoon kosher or sea salt

¼ teaspoon black pepper

Whether it's a few extra spinach leaves or the remnants in a bag of frozen broccoli, Serena's favorite trick for using up bits of leftover veggies is to make this cheese, egg, and bread dish. She usually adds about 1½ cups total of any type of chopped vegetables to her strata. In this version, we use canned artichokes because we think they should be in every Mediterranean pantry for their flavor, nutrition, and convenience. Leftover pita bread gives a Greek twist to this versatile recipe.

Spread the pita bread pieces on a large rimmed baking sheet and place it into the cold oven. Heat the oven to 400°F. Remove the toasted bread from the oven after 6 to 7 minutes or when toasted. Place the baking sheet on a wire rack to cool for 3 minutes to allow the bread to crisp.

Spray a 9×13-inch metal baking pan with cooking spray. Arrange the artichoke quarters evenly in the pan.

In a large bowl, whisk together the eggs, milk, ½ cup of the cheese, the dill, salt, and pepper. Gently mix the slightly cooled pita bread into the egg mixture, then pour into the prepared baking pan. Sprinkle the remaining ½ cup cheese evenly over the top of the strata.

Bake for 18 to 20 minutes, until the center is just set. (Avoid overbaking, as the strata will continue to cook after you remove it from the oven.) Serve warm or at room temperature.

Healthy Kitchen Hack: We use a metal pan for this recipe to save some time in the oven, as metal heats up more quickly than glass. If you prefer to use a glass casserole dish, add an additional 5 to 7 minutes to the baking time.

Per Serving: Calories: 276; Total Fat: 12g; Saturated Fat: 6g; Cholesterol: 208mg; Sodium: 597mg; Total Carbohydrates: 25g; Fiber: 4g; Protein: 16g

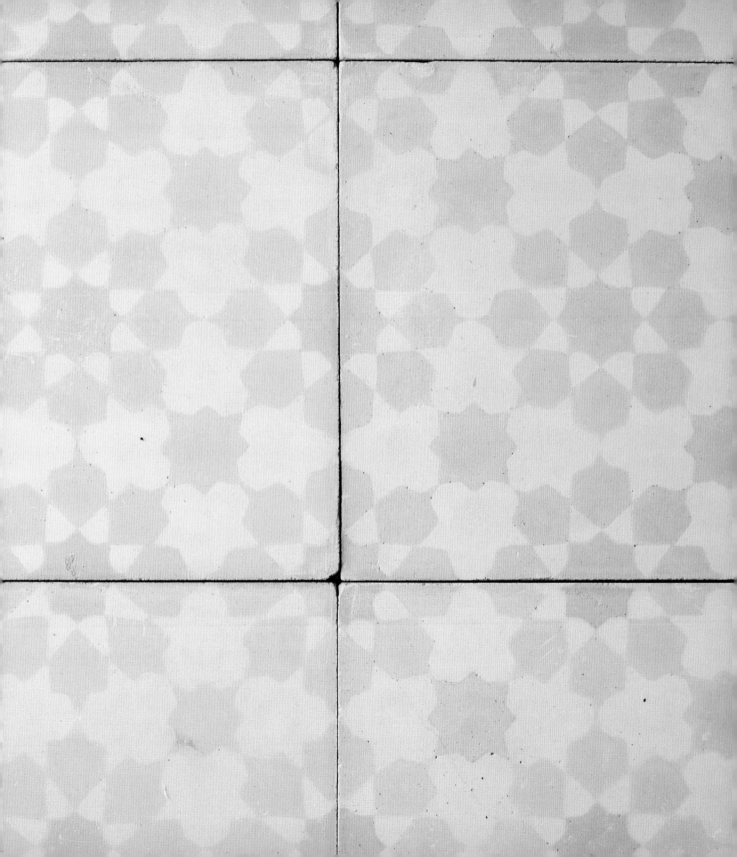

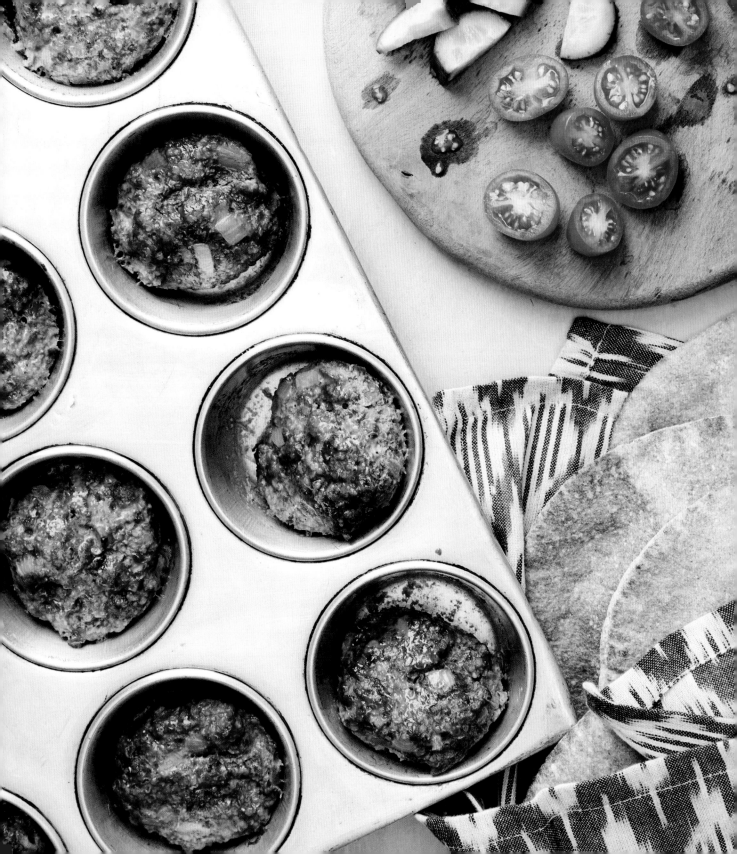

meat

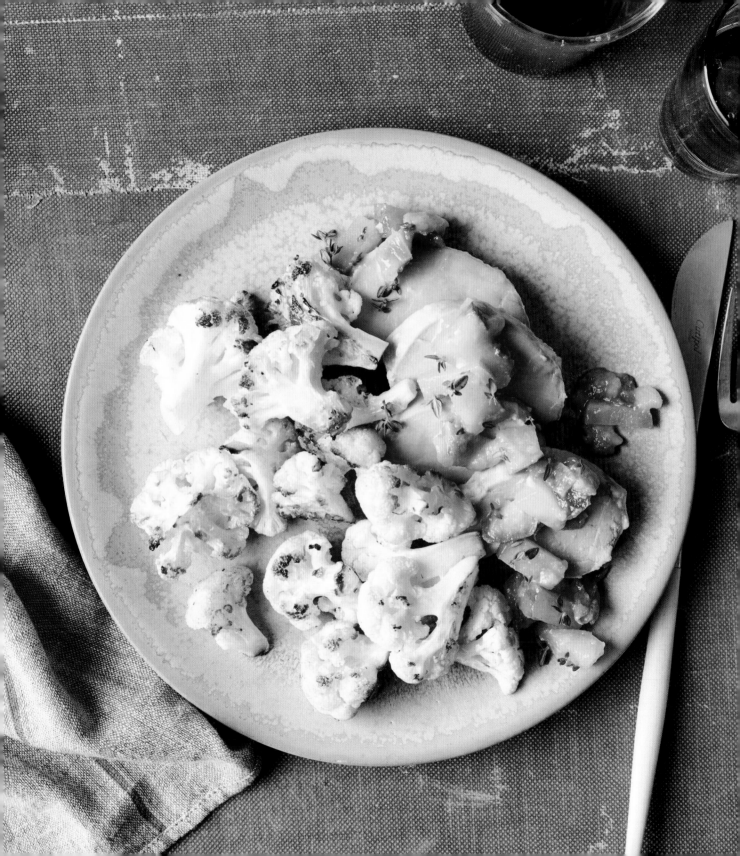

Roasted Pork Tenderloin with Cauliflower and Pears

| Nut-Free, Gluten-Free, Egg-Free | Serves 4 | Prep time: 15 minutes | Cook time: 20 minutes |

1 pork tenderloin (about 1 pound)

1 small head cauliflower (about 1 pound)

½ cup plain 2% Greek yogurt (about 4 ounces)

2 tablespoons extra-virgin olive oil, divided

¾ teaspoon kosher or sea salt, divided

¼ cup chopped red onion

2 pears, cored and chopped (about 2 cups)

1 tablespoon honey

1 tablespoon white wine vinegar or rice vinegar

1 teaspoon chopped fresh thyme leaves

In the Ball household, this recipe received the highest rating in the book: thumbs-up from everyone and a few "Mom, why don't you *always* make cauliflower like this?" Even the cousins visiting from Michigan (Serena doubled the recipe) were surprised that pork tenderloin—a low-saturated-fat cut of meat—could be so juicy and tender. Our secret to keeping any lean meat from drying out during cooking is to slather it with our Olive Oil–Yogurt Spread (page 42) as we do here.

Preheat the oven to 450°F. Line a large rimmed baking sheet with aluminum foil and coat it with cooking spray. Place the pork on the lined baking sheet.

Cut the cauliflower into florets of about 1 inch. Coarsely cut up the cauliflower leaves and slice the stem into ½-inch-thick rounds. Place all the prepped cauliflower into a large bowl.

Into a medium bowl, measure the yogurt, 1 tablespoon of the olive oil, and ½ teaspoon of the salt. Whisk to combine. Scoop out half of the yogurt mixture and add to the cauliflower bowl; toss to combine.

Using your hands or a rubber scraper, spread the remaining yogurt mixture on all sides of the pork. Spread out the cauliflower on the baking sheet around and on top of the pork so there is as much room as possible for heat to circulate around the cauliflower.

Roast for 10 minutes. Remove from the oven, stir the cauliflower, and flip the pork over. Roast for 5 to 10 more minutes (depending on the weight of the pork) until the internal temperature measures 140°F on a meat thermometer. Remove from the oven and let the pork rest for about 5 minutes until the internal temperature measures 145°F. Reserve the cooking juices on the baking sheet and transfer the pork to a cutting board. Slice the pork, place on a serving platter, and add the cauliflower.

continued

While the pork is cooking, heat the remaining 1 tablespoon olive oil in a medium saucepan over medium heat. Add the onion and cook, stirring occasionally, until golden, about 5 minutes. Add the pears and cook, stirring occasionally, for 3 more minutes.

Carefully scrape the cooking juices from the baking sheet into the saucepan and then add the honey, vinegar, thyme, remaining ¼ teaspoon salt, and 2 tablespoons water. Cook until most of the liquid has evaporated, 4 to 5 minutes. Stir and serve the pear sauce with the pork and cauliflower.

Healthy Kitchen Hack: To avoid hidden salt, look for pork tenderloin or chicken that hasn't been marinated or injected with a solution to keep it "tender and juicy." Avoid labels with the words "marinated in" or "added solution." Without these additions, the true pork or chicken flavor will shine through in your dish while keeping the sodium in check. If you can't find pork or chicken without these words, cut the amount of salt in your recipe in half.

Per Serving: Calories: 297; Total Fat: 11g; Saturated Fat: 2g; Cholesterol: 77mg; Sodium: 465mg; Total Carbohydrates: 22g; Fiber: 5g; Protein: 29g

Pepper-and-Sausage Skillet Supper

Dairy-Free, Nut-Free, Gluten-Free, Egg-Free	Serves 4	Prep time: 5 minutes	Cook time: 30 minutes

1 tablespoon extra-virgin olive oil

1 large yellow or white onion, chopped

2 garlic cloves, minced

½ teaspoon dried thyme

⅛ teaspoon crushed red pepper

12 ounces hot or sweet Italian sausage links, cut into 1-inch pieces

1½ cups uncooked instant brown rice

1 tablespoon tomato paste

¼ teaspoon black pepper

1 (12-ounce) jar roasted red peppers or 2 Roasted Red Peppers (page 44), sliced into strips

⅓ cup torn fresh basil leaves

When you're craving traditional Italian-style sausage and peppers, turn to this recipe. Here we pair spicy sausage with whole grains, extra veggies, and fresh herbs as a way to extend the meat while loading up with some extra nutrients. Cooking the rice along with all the other ingredients means one less pot you'll be cleaning post-meal. We like to pair this with a bowl of mixed greens like our Arugula with Apricot Balsamic Dressing (page 62) or our Herb Salad with Citrus-Date Dressing (page 73).

In a large skillet over medium heat, heat the olive oil. Add the onion and cook, stirring often, for 4 minutes. Add the garlic, thyme, and crushed red pepper. Cook, stirring frequently, for 1 minute. Add the sausage pieces and cook, stirring occasionally, for 3 minutes (the sausage will not be cooked through).

Increase the heat to medium-high. Add the rice and 3½ cups water to the skillet; bring to a boil. Once boiling, reduce the heat to medium-low, cover the skillet, and cook for 15 minutes.

Stir in the tomato paste and black pepper until incorporated. Add the roasted peppers, stir, and cook until heated through, 1 to 2 minutes. Remove from the stove and sprinkle with the basil. Serve from the skillet.

Healthy Kitchen Hack: If you already have cooked whole grains on hand, such as leftover rice, couscous, barley, or quinoa, use in place of the uncooked instant brown rice. Follow the recipe directions but cook the sausage for 10 minutes (instead of 3 minutes). Mix in about 4 cups of your chosen cooked whole grain and ¾ cup water along with the tomato paste, salt, and black pepper (add a few more tablespoons of water if not "saucy" enough). Finish with the roasted peppers and basil as directed.

Per Serving: Calories: 471; Total Fat: 27g; Saturated Fat: 9g; Cholesterol: 62mg; Sodium: 939mg; Total Carbohydrates: 43g; Fiber: 2g; Protein: 18g

Flat Iron Steak, Onions, and Tomatoes over Hummus

| Dairy-Free, Egg-Free | Serves 4 | Prep time: 10 minutes | Cook time: 10 minutes |

2 tablespoons extra-virgin olive oil

1 tablespoon red wine vinegar

2 teaspoons dried oregano

½ teaspoon kosher or sea salt

¼ teaspoon black pepper

1 pint grape tomatoes

1 red onion, cut into ¾-inch wedges keeping root end on, so wedges stay intact

1 pound boneless flat iron steak, about ¾ inch thick (for similar cuts, see headnote)

1 (10-ounce) container hummus or homemade hummus (see Healthy Kitchen Hack on page 50)

2 (6-inch) whole-wheat pita breads, cut into eighths

Flat iron steak is one of the most underrated cuts of meat you can buy. It delivers rich, beefy flavor and top-notch texture, but at a fraction of the price of flank or skirt steak. Depending on where you live, you may see similar cuts of meat also called hanger, sirloin tip, bavette, or flap steaks. These thin, relatively lean cuts are also best when quick-cooked on the grill or under the broiler. We're also big fans of our broilers to add sweet caramelized flavor and a bit of char to veggies (as in this recipe) along with speeding up the cooking time of beef. Because every oven is different, be sure to get to know your own broiler and use our range of broiling times to your advantage (versus a "burnt to a crisp" disaster!).

Place one oven rack 3 to 4 inches below the broiler. Preheat the broiler to high for 10 minutes. Line a large rimmed baking sheet with aluminum foil and place a wire rack on the foil. Coat with cooking spray.

Into a large bowl, put the olive oil, vinegar, oregano, salt, and black pepper and whisk to combine. Add the tomatoes and onion; toss well to coat. Using a slotted spoon or your hands (so most of the olive oil mixture remains in the bowl), place the vegetables around the edges of the wire rack (leaving room in the middle for the steak). Place the steak in the bowl. Rub both sides of the meat to coat with the remaining olive oil mixture. Place the steak in the center of the wire rack. Fold under the thinner end of the steak to ensure even cooking.

Broil the steak and vegetables for 5 minutes. Remove from the oven and, using tongs, flip the steak and turn any vegetables that have started to darken. Place the steak and vegetables back under the broiler. Broil until the internal temperature of the steak measures 135° to 140°F on a meat thermometer, another 4 to 6 minutes. (*Watch closely* to avoid completely charred vegetables.

See the Healthy Kitchen Hack on page 237 for information on meat cooking temperatures; you may want to cook only to 120°F to 130°F.) Remove the steak to a cutting board and cover loosely with foil; let rest for 5 minutes until the internal temperature reaches 145°F.

Spread the hummus on a serving platter and top with the roasted vegetables. (If using our hummus recipe, spread half of the batch on the platter and store the remainder in the refrigerator for a future use.)

Slice the steak thinly across the grain and place on top of the vegetables and hummus. Serve with the pita bread.

Healthy Kitchen Hack: Quick-cooking flat iron, flap, and hanger steaks are also excellent for grilling. Transfer this recipe to the grill by placing the coated vegetables on a large piece of heavy-duty aluminum foil or in a grilling basket coated with cooking spray. Grill uncovered for 3 to 4 minutes over high heat. Grill the steak on a grill grate coated with cooking spray for 3 minutes on one side and 2 to 3 minutes on the other side until it reaches the desired doneness.

Per Serving: Calories: 443; Total Fat: 21g; Saturated Fat: 5g; Cholesterol: 66mg; Sodium: 596mg; Total Carbohydrates: 33g; Fiber: 8g; Protein: 34g

"The finished meal looked great—especially next to my bright green salad. I admit, I thought the hummus would be weird with steak, but it totally worked and was delightful! This dish goes wonderfully with a glass of red wine."

—Wendy from Arvada, CO

The Best Baked Italian Meatballs

Dairy-Free, Nut-Free, Gluten-Free | Serves 4 | Prep time: 10 minutes | Cook time: 20 minutes

4 garlic cloves

½ teaspoon kosher or sea salt

1 pound 80% to 90% lean ground beef

⅓ cup panko breadcrumbs

1 large egg

1 tablespoon dried oregano

¼ teaspoon black pepper

We think this will become your new go-to meatball recipe. Serena tinkered with and cooked this recipe three nights in a row and then her kids asked her to make it a fourth night! To keep these lean meatballs juicy, use a gentle touch as you combine the ingredients, being careful not to overmix. Serve your new favorite meatballs over plates of pasta, in meatball sandwiches, or on top of grain bowls.

Preheat the oven to 400°F. Line a large rimmed baking sheet with parchment paper or aluminum foil.

Slice the garlic cloves and then sprinkle the salt over the slices. Mince the garlic slices together with the salt; the cutting motion will mix them together and turn them into a rough paste.

Into a large bowl, put the garlic mixture, ground beef, breadcrumbs, egg, oregano, and black pepper. Using your hands, gently mix the ingredients together. Divide the meat into 16 (1-ounce) portions. Shape each portion into a 1½-inch meatball. Place them on the prepared baking sheet.

Bake for 15 to 17 minutes until the internal temperature of the meatballs measures 160°F on a meat thermometer. Serve immediately or store in the freezer in a freezer bag for up to 3 months.

Healthy Kitchen Hack: Turn these meatballs into kebabs! But instead of grilling them (turning them on the grill can be tricky), use your oven. Thread metal or wooden (no need to soak in water) skewers with a combination of grape tomatoes and meatballs. We suggest this order: tomato—meatball—2 tomatoes—meatball—tomato. Bake as directed above and serve over rice or couscous with torn fresh basil leaves.

Per Serving: Calories: 236; Total Fat: 11g; Saturated Fat: 4g; Cholesterol: 121mg; Sodium: 329mg; Total Carbohydrates: 7g; Fiber: 1g; Protein: 25g

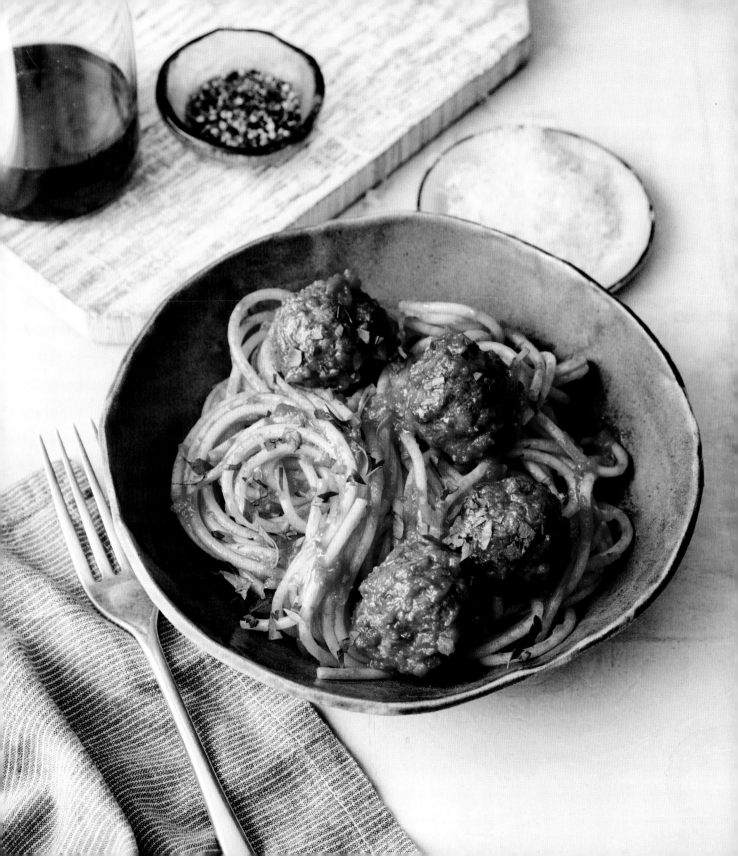

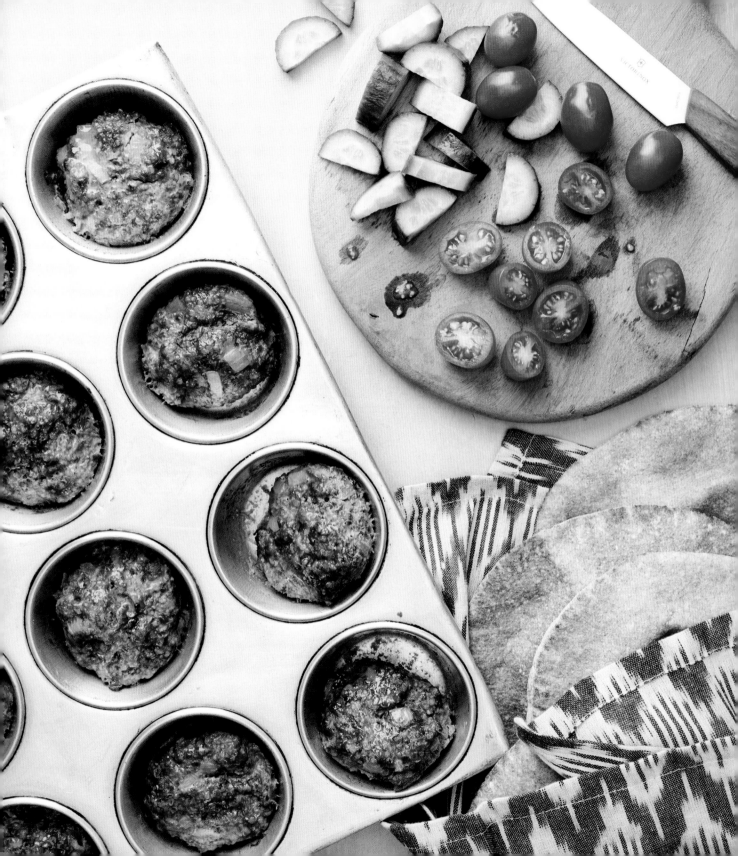

Beef and Quinoa Koftas

Dairy-Free, Nut-Free, Gluten-Free	Serves 4	Prep time: 10 minutes	Cook time: 35 minutes

⅓ cup uncooked quinoa

2 teaspoons extra-virgin olive oil

½ cup finely minced onion (about ¼ onion)

½ teaspoon garlic powder

½ teaspoon kosher or sea salt

¼ teaspoon ground cinnamon

¼ teaspoon ground cumin

¼ teaspoon black pepper

¼ teaspoon crushed red pepper

1 pound 80% to 90% lean ground beef or lamb

1 large egg

Sliced tomatoes, sliced cucumbers, and pita bread, for serving (optional)

In the Middle East, spiced mini meatloaves known as koftas reign supreme—from Turkey, where ground lamb, beef, or chicken are combined with dried fruits and spices like cinnamon and cumin, to finger-shaped Egyptian koftas, to those on Cyprus which combine meat with lentils or bulgur. We find shaping koftas in muffin pans is quick and faster to bake than a full-size meatloaf. And after doing lots of yummy research, Serena discovered that cooked quinoa not only extends the ground beef but also helps keep the koftas from drying out.

Preheat the oven to 400°F. Coat a 12-cup muffin tin with cooking spray.

Place the quinoa in a fine-mesh strainer and hold under cold running water until water runs clear; drain well.

In a medium saucepan, bring 1 cup water to a boil. Add the quinoa. Reduce the heat to low and cover. Cook until the germ spirals out from the grain, about 15 minutes. Drain any remaining water. Spread on a plate to cool slightly.

While the quinoa is cooking, in a medium skillet over medium heat, heat the olive oil. Add the onion and cook, stirring, until translucent, 4 to 5 minutes. Remove from the heat and set aside.

In a large bowl, stir together the garlic powder, salt, cinnamon, cumin, black pepper, and crushed red pepper. Add the beef, egg, cooked quinoa, and cooked onion. Using your hands, gently mix the ingredients together. (Do not overwork the meat or it will become tough.) Divide the beef mixture into 12 portions and place in the prepared muffin cups. Bake for 16 to 18 minutes until the internal temperature of the koftas measures 160°F on a meat thermometer.

Serve with tomatoes, cucumbers, and pita bread, if desired.

continued

Beef and Quinoa Koftas (continued)

Healthy Kitchen Hack: To make these mini meatloaves even more juicy—and more "authentically" Middle Eastern—add ¼ cup diced prunes (6 to 7 prunes) to the meat mixture.

Per Serving (koftas only): Calories: 268; Total Fat: 11g; Saturated Fat: 4g; Cholesterol: 75mg; Sodium: 302mg; Total Carbohydrates: 17g; Fiber: 1g; Protein: 25g

"My boys do lots of winter sports, so they need healthy food to fuel them. Even with the new combo of spices, the boys gave these two thumbs up!"

—Erin from Bottineau, ND

Loaded Mini Burgers on Grilled Sweet Potatoes

Nut-Free, Gluten-Free, Egg-Free	Serves 4	Prep time: 15 minutes	Cook time: 10 minutes

2 cups sliced white mushrooms

1 pound 80% to 90% lean ground beef

1 teaspoon Worcestershire sauce or less-sodium soy sauce

½ teaspoon garlic powder

¼ teaspoon kosher or sea salt

¼ teaspoon black pepper

3 medium sweet potatoes, unpeeled, sliced into ½-inch thick rounds

2 teaspoons extra-virgin olive oil

8 cracker-size pieces light cheddar cheese (2 ounces)

1 avocado, halved, pit removed

2 tomatoes, sliced into quarters

8 lettuce leaves

We considered calling these "Flavor Bomb Sliders." Not only are they stacked a mile high with veggies (the Mediterranean way to eat a burger) but the beef is also enriched with savory, meaty mushrooms. Budget-friendly humble white mushrooms provide volume, nutrition, and deliciousness—they also have umami, which is a "savoriness" or "meatiness" that makes your mouth water as these sliders do.

Coat a cold grill with cooking spray and heat to medium-high.

Put half of the mushrooms into a food processor and pulse about 15 times, until the mushrooms are finely chopped but not pureed, similar to the texture of ground meat. Remove and place in a medium bowl. Repeat with the remaining mushrooms.

To the bowl with the mushrooms, add the ground beef, Worcestershire sauce, garlic powder, salt, and black pepper. Using your hands, gently mix the ingredients together. Divide the meat into 8 equal portions. Shape each portion into a burger about ½ inch thick. Gently press your thumb into the center of each burger to make a ¼-inch-deep indentation (to ensure the center cooks evenly). Place the burgers on a plate and set aside.

Brush both sides of the sweet potatoes with the olive oil.

Once the grill is hot, place the burgers on one half of the grill and the sweet potatoes on the other half. Cook the burgers, flipping halfway through with a metal spatula, until the internal temperature is 160°F on a meat thermometer, 6 to 8 minutes total. During the last minute of cooking, top with the cheese.

Cook the sweet potatoes, flipping halfway through with metal tongs, until they just start to soften (do not overcook), 8 to 10 minutes total.

Place each slider on a slice of sweet potato. Scoop out one-eighth of the avocado and "smash" it on top of each burger. Top evenly with the tomato slices and lettuce. Place the remaining sweet potato slices on top of each burger to make a "bun" and serve.

continued

Loaded Mini Burgers on Grilled Sweet Potatoes (continued)

Healthy Kitchen Hack: You can use a broiler instead of the grill for this recipe. Line a large rimmed baking sheet with aluminum foil. Broil the burgers and the sweet potatoes, flipping halfway through and arranging so they brown evenly. The broiling times will be about the same as the grilling times—but you will need to remove the burgers from the oven before the sweet potatoes are done; return the sweet potatoes to the oven to finish cooking.

Per Serving: Calories: 393; Total Fat: 18g; Saturated Fat: 5g; Cholesterol: 75mg; Sodium: 270mg; Total Carbohydrates: 32g; Fiber: 8g; Protein: 27g

"These sliders looked impressive and tasted delicious! I used a cast iron grill skillet instead of a grill and it worked great. Next time I'll try them with blue cheese."

—Sara from Storrs, CT

Steak with Salted Roast Potatoes

Dairy-Free, Nut-Free, Gluten-Free, Egg-Free	Serves 6	Prep time: 5 minutes	Cook time: 35 minutes

1½ pounds red potatoes, cut into 1-inch cubes

1 medium lemon

2 tablespoons extra-virgin olive oil, divided

1 teaspoon crushed dried oregano

½ teaspoon plus ⅛ teaspoon kosher or sea salt, divided

½ teaspoon black pepper, divided

1½ pounds boneless sirloin or top sirloin steak (about ¾ inch thick)

Traditionally, most people cook steak by searing it in a pan first and then roasting in the oven. We do the opposite for two reasons: Oven-roasting heats the steak slowly to keep the proteins from seizing up quickly and getting tough. Also, more of the saturated fat can drip out of the steak as it's warmed gently. At the end, a quick pan sear makes a beautiful brown crust. While this isn't an everyday Mediterranean Diet dish, please enjoy it leisurely with friends; that *is* the Mediterranean way.

Place one oven rack in the middle of the oven and another rack in the top half of the oven. Place a large rimmed baking sheet on either oven rack. Preheat the oven to 400°F.

Put the potatoes in a large bowl. Grate the lemon zest with a Microplane or citrus zester over the potatoes. Reserve the zested lemon. Add 1 tablespoon of the oil, the oregano, ½ teaspoon of the salt, and the black pepper to the bowl. Toss to combine.

Carefully remove the hot baking sheet from the oven and coat with cooking spray. Add the potatoes to the baking sheet and spread out. Roast on the middle rack for 15 minutes. Reduce the oven temperature to 300°F and carefully remove the baking sheet to stir the potatoes. Place the potatoes back in the oven and roast for another 15 to 17 minutes, until just fork-tender.

While the potatoes cook, line a second large rimmed baking sheet with foil and place a wire rack on the foil; coat with cooking spray. Place the steak on the rack and sprinkle with the remaining ⅛ teaspoon salt. After the oven has been reduced to 300°F and at the same time the potatoes go back into the oven, place the steak on the top oven rack and cook for 15 to 17 minutes until the internal temperature measures 100°F on a meat thermometer.

When the steak is about 5 minutes away from being done in the oven, place a cast iron skillet over medium-high heat for 3 minutes. Add the remaining 1 tablespoon oil and heat for about 2 minutes more.

continued

Remove the steak from the oven and place it in the hot oil in the skillet. Cook the steak until it develops a brown crust, about 1 minute. Flip using large tongs. Cook the other side until it develops a brown crust and the internal temperature measures 135° to 140°F on a meat thermometer, 1 to 3 minutes. (See the Healthy Kitchen Hack below.) Remove the steak to a cutting board and cover loosely with foil; let rest for 5 minutes until the internal temperature reaches 145°F. Cut into 6 steaks.

Cut the reserved lemon in half and squeeze 2 tablespoons of the juice over the potatoes. (Save any remaining lemon for another use.) Serve the potatoes with the steaks.

Healthy Kitchen Hack: A chef will tell you that the correct internal cooking temperature of a medium-rare steak is 120°F and a medium-well steak is 130°F. As dietitians wearing our food safety hats, we say a steak should not be eaten below 145°F. However, steak is rarely a cause of foodborne illness and we know that people don't like overcooked steak. If you are diligent with keeping your meat refrigerated after you purchase it, you are not serving anyone with a compromised immune system, and you're certain your meat thermometer is accurate, refer to the chef temperatures for how well-done you like your steak.

Per Serving: Calories: 266; Total Fat: 9g; Saturated Fat: 2g; Cholesterol: 65mg; Sodium: 273mg; Total Carbohydrates: 19g; Fiber: 2g; Protein: 27g

Greek Sloppy Yos

Dairy-Free, Nut-Free, Egg-Free		Serves 4	Prep time: 10 minutes	Cook time: 20 minutes

1 tablespoon extra-virgin olive oil

3 celery stalks, diced

½ bell pepper, any color, diced

¼ large red or yellow onion, diced

2 garlic cloves, minced

1 pound 90% lean ground beef

2 teaspoons dried oregano

¼ teaspoon kosher or sea salt

¼ teaspoon black pepper

1 (15-ounce) can cannellini beans, drained and rinsed

1 cup low-sodium tomato sauce or Easy Roasted Tomato Sauce (page 147)

2 tablespoons ketchup

2 tablespoons honey

2 teaspoons Worcestershire sauce or less-sodium soy sauce

1 teaspoon red wine vinegar

3 (7- or 8-inch) whole-wheat pita breads, cut in half

2 English seedless cucumbers, chopped

4 lettuce leaves

Our Mediterranean twist on the classic messy meat sandwich features one of our favorite ground meat extenders: beans! Creamy, mild cannellini beans practically melt into this seasoned, tomatoey beef mixture, adding extra fiber, vitamins, and minerals incognito. This recipe is our top recommendation to get your favorite meat lovers into eating more plant foods. (It's up to you if you want to share your secret ingredient or not!)

In a large skillet over medium heat, heat the olive oil. Add the celery, bell pepper, and onion and cook for 4 minutes, stirring occasionally. Add the garlic and cook for 1 minute, stirring frequently. Add the ground beef, oregano, salt, and black pepper. Break up the meat with a wooden spoon and cook, stirring occasionally, until the beef is no longer pink, 8 to 10 minutes.

While the beef cooks, add the beans to a large bowl. Using a potato masher or a fork, mash the beans until they resemble a puree or paste. Set aside.

To the skillet with the meat, add the tomato sauce, ketchup, honey, Worcestershire sauce, and vinegar. Mix until everything is incorporated. Add the beans and mix in thoroughly. With a wooden spoon, mash and stir in any beans that are still whole and cook until the sauce is heated through, 2 to 3 minutes.

To serve, stuff the meat, chopped cucumber, and lettuce leaves into the 6 pita bread halves.

Healthy Kitchen Hack: This beef mix makes for a fantastic pasta sauce; or use the leftovers as a topping for baked potatoes for a quickie dinner.

Per Serving: Calories: 358; Total Fat: 11g; Saturated Fat: 3g; Cholesterol: 49mg; Sodium: 487mg; Total Carbohydrates: 44g; Fiber: 8g; Protein: 24g

One-Pot Lamb with Olives and Mushrooms

Dairy-Free, Nut-Free, Gluten-Free, Egg-Free	Serves 4	Prep time: 5 minutes	Cook time: 40 minutes

1 pound bone-in or boneless lamb leg steak, center cut

1 tablespoon extra-virgin olive oil

¼ teaspoon kosher or sea salt

¼ teaspoon black pepper

½ medium yellow or white onion, chopped

1 large green or red bell pepper, chopped

¾ teaspoon smoked paprika

2 cups sliced mushrooms

2 garlic cloves, chopped

⅓ cup dry red wine

1 (15-ounce) can crushed tomatoes

1 (8-ounce) jar green or black olives, drained and rinsed

Per Serving (without couscous):
Calories: 297; Total Fat: 14g; Saturated Fat: 3g; Cholesterol: 65mg; Sodium: 681mg; Total Carbohydrates: 20g; Fiber: 6g; Protein: 25g

As we do with all our soups and stews, we've included steps to bring out the best in all the flavors—it adds a few minutes to the cook time, but it's worth it! French chefs have done this for centuries by creating classic "mother sauces" like espagnole sauce, the inspiration for this recipe. We use lamb, a popular Mediterranean meat, to make a thick, saucy stew so good you'll be licking the spoon. If you wish, serve over couscous.

Trim the fat off the edges of the lamb and cut the meat into 1-inch cubes, including a cube with the small bone. (That small piece of bone adds terrific flavor and nutrients to the dish!) Pat the cubes dry with paper towels.

In a large stockpot over medium-high heat, heat the olive oil. Add the lamb (including the bone-in piece), salt, and black pepper. Cook, without stirring, until one side of the meat is browned, about 5 minutes. Using tongs, remove the meat to a plate. (The meat will still be pink in places.)

To the same pot, add the onion, bell pepper, and smoked paprika. Cook, stirring occasionally, for 8 minutes. Push the onion mixture to the sides of the pot, then add the mushrooms and garlic. Cook, stirring occasionally, until most of the liquid released by the mushrooms has evaporated, 5 to 6 minutes. Add the wine and 1 cup water. Cook, scraping up the browned pieces on the bottom of the pot, for 3 minutes. Add the tomatoes, lamb, and any lamb juices that have accumulated on the plate. Bring to a boil, then reduce the heat to medium and cook until the stew thickens, 10 to 15 minutes. Add the olives and stir. Cook for 1 minute, until heated through.

Healthy Kitchen Hack: Don't toss those mushrooms you forgot about in the fridge—ones that have browned and are slightly shriveled actually have a meatier flavor. To perfectly "age" mushrooms, refrigerate them sealed in their package and avoid storing in the crisper drawer.

Spanish Ham and Beans

Dairy-Free, Nut-Free, Egg-Free	Serves 6	Prep time: 5 minutes	Cook time: 25 minutes

2 tablespoons extra-virgin olive oil

½ medium yellow or white onion

1 large green or red bell pepper, sliced into 2-inch strips

1 teaspoon ground turmeric

¼ teaspoon black pepper

1½ cups diced cooked ham (6 ounces)

4 garlic cloves, minced

¼ cup dry white wine

2 cups low-sodium chicken broth

2 tablespoons tomato paste

1 (15-ounce) can pinto beans, drained and rinsed

1½ cups chopped fresh parsley, divided

1½ cups uncooked couscous (from a 6-ounce box)

⅓ cup sliced green olives

If there's a one-pot meal that embodies the Mediterranean Diet, this is it. While we call this stovetop dish "Spanish," it could easily be Italian, Moroccan, Turkish, etc. The basic formula is abundant vegetables, beans, a whole grain, olive oil, olives, lots of herbs, spices, and a bit of meat for flavoring. We encourage you to use this recipe template as a starting point to expand your culinary horizons using your Mediterranean pantry.

In a large stockpot over medium-high heat, heat the olive oil. Add the onion, bell pepper, turmeric, and black pepper and cook, stirring occasionally, for 8 minutes. Push the onion mixture to the sides of the pot and add the ham. Cook, without stirring, until the ham begins to brown, about 3 minutes. Push the ham to the side of the pot and add the garlic; stir constantly for 1 minute. Pour in the wine and cook until most of the liquid evaporates, 1 to 2 minutes. Increase the heat to high and add the broth, 1 cup water, the tomato paste, beans, and 1 cup of the parsley; bring to a boil. Stir in the couscous, cover the pot, and turn off the heat. Let the couscous absorb the liquid for 5 minutes. Remove the lid and stir in the remaining ½ cup parsley and the olives.

Healthy Kitchen Hack: To make this recipe even more budget-friendly, cook the beans from scratch with a ham bone. Follow the instructions above, adding a cooked ham bone or ham hock to the pot instead of the ham. Then instead of canned beans, add 1 cup dried pinto beans (soaked overnight), 1 cup uncooked brown rice, and enough water to cover the contents of the pot by at least 2 inches. Cover the pot and bring to boil over medium-high heat, then reduce the heat to low and simmer until tender, 2 to 3 hours. Stir in all the parsley and the olives, then serve.

Per Serving: Calories: 301; Total Fat: 9g; Saturated Fat: 2g; Cholesterol: 18mg; Sodium: 537mg; Total Carbohydrates: 40g; Fiber: 4g; Protein: 14g

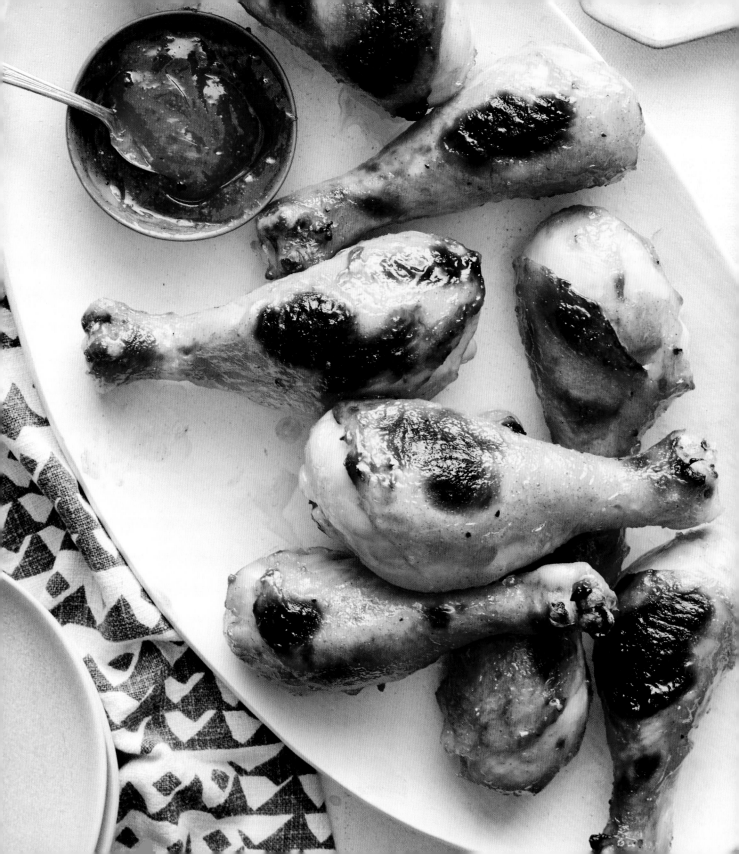

poultry

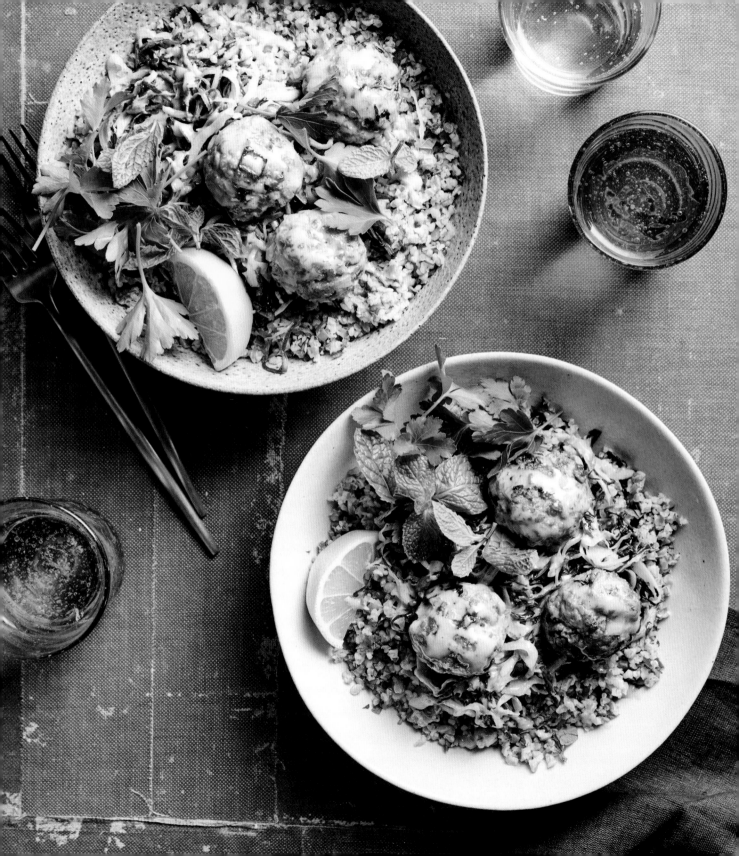

Turkey Meatball Grain Bowls with Honey-Tahini Sauce

| Dairy-Free, Nut-Free, Egg-Free | Serves 6 | Prep time: 15 minutes | Cook time: 15 minutes |

1 (10-ounce) package cabbage slaw mix or broccoli slaw (about 6 cups)

4 tablespoons extra-virgin olive oil, divided

1 pound 93% lean ground turkey

3 cups cooked bulgur, divided

¼ cup diced onion

¼ cup chopped fresh parsley

4 tablespoons chopped fresh mint leaves, divided

2 garlic cloves, minced

½ teaspoon kosher or sea salt, divided

1 medium lemon, cut in half

¼ cup tahini

1½ tablespoons honey

We love all the ingredient tricks that can extend ground meat into more servings without sacrificing taste. Here we use bulgur, cracked wheat that's a staple whole grain in Mediterranean cuisine. It cooks up in less than 15 minutes. And wait until you taste the honey-tahini sauce—let's just say it's Deanna's new favorite condiment (see more in the Healthy Kitchen Hack below).

Position the oven racks in the middle and upper half of the oven. Preheat the oven to 375°F. Line a large rimmed baking sheet with parchment paper or aluminum foil.

On a second large rimmed baking sheet, put the slaw mix and 3 tablespoons of the olive oil. Toss together with your hands. Spread the coated slaw out evenly and set aside.

In a large bowl, put the ground turkey, ½ cup of the cooked bulgur, the onion, parsley, 2 tablespoons of the mint, the garlic, and ¼ teaspoon of the salt. Using your hands, gently mix the ingredients together and evenly shape the mixture into 18 (1½-inch) meatballs. Place them on the foil-lined baking sheet. Brush the meatballs with the remaining 1 tablespoon olive oil. Bake for 12 to 15 minutes until the middle of the meatballs tests 165°F with a meat thermometer. Bake the slaw for 15 minutes, mixing halfway through.

Squeeze 2 tablespoons of lemon juice into a blender or a food processor, reserving the rest of the lemon. Add the tahini, honey, and 2 tablespoons water. Blend until smooth. Add more water, 1 tablespoon at a time, until the sauce is a thick but pourable consistency. Set aside.

Squeeze 1 tablespoon of lemon juice into a large bowl. (Save any remaining lemon for another use.) Add the remaining 2½ cups cooked bulgur, 2 tablespoons mint, and ¼ teaspoon salt. Add about a quarter of the tahini sauce and mix all the ingredients together.

continued

In another bowl, mix the cooked slaw and another quarter of the tahini sauce.

To serve, divide the bulgur mix among six bowls. Top with the slaw and 3 meatballs for each bowl. Drizzle with the remaining honey-tahini sauce.

Healthy Kitchen Hack: This magical honey-tahini sauce is fantastic with both savory dishes—like this recipe—and sweet treats. Omit a few tablespoons of water and serve it as a dip with raw vegetables and toasted pita. For desserts, try it as topping over fresh fruit or see how we use it as an icing for our Tahini Brownies (page 269).

Per Serving: Calories: 372; Total Fat: 21g; Saturated Fat: 4g; Cholesterol: 52mg; Sodium: 230mg; Total Carbohydrates: 30g; Fiber: 7g; Protein: 21g

Smoked Paprika Chicken over Roasted Pepper–Corn Salad

Dairy-Free, Nut-Free, Gluten-Free, Egg-Free	Serves 6	Prep time: 15 minutes	Cook time: 15 minutes

1 medium red onion, cut into quarters

1½ pounds boneless, skinless chicken breasts, cut into 6 portions

1 carrot, cut into 4 pieces

1 celery stalk, cut into 4 pieces

¾ teaspoon kosher or sea salt, divided

½ cup chopped fresh cilantro

2 tablespoons extra-virgin olive oil

1 tablespoon orange juice

1 lime, cut in half

1½ teaspoons honey

¼ teaspoon black pepper

2 cups thawed frozen corn kernels, or kernels from 3 cooked corncobs

1 (12-ounce) jar roasted red peppers, drained and chopped, or 2 Roasted Red Peppers (page 44), drained and diced

2 avocados, pitted, peeled, and chopped

¾ teaspoon smoked paprika, divided

Bring some spice and color into your weekday dinner routine with this no-fuss but flavorful chicken dish. Poaching chicken is a great way to keep the meat juicy while not having to keep an eye on it while it's cooking. The roasted pepper–corn salad is fantastic in the summertime when fresh corn is at its peak. Summer is also a great time to switch this up by prepping the vegetables on the grill.

Dice one of the onion quarters (you should end up with about ½ cup). Set aside.

Place the three remaining onion quarters into a medium saucepan. Add the chicken, carrots, and celery. Fill the pan with water until the chicken is submerged by 1 inch. Add ½ teaspoon of the salt. Place the pan over medium-high heat and bring to a boil. Once boiling, reduce the heat to medium-low, cover with a lid, and cook until the internal temperature of the largest piece of chicken measures 165°F with a meat thermometer, 12 to 15 minutes. Remove the chicken from the water and let it rest for 5 minutes on a cutting board. Strain the liquid and save for another use (see the Healthy Kitchen Hack on page 248).

In a blender or food processor, add the cilantro, olive oil, orange juice, juice from half the lime, honey, the remaining ¼ teaspoon salt, and the black pepper. Process until completely smooth.

In a large bowl, add the corn, roasted peppers, avocado, the reserved diced onion, and ½ teaspoon of the smoked paprika. Mix well. Pour in about half of the cilantro dressing and mix again.

To serve, spread the roasted pepper–corn salad on the bottom of a serving platter. Top with the chicken. Sprinkle with the remaining ¼ teaspoon smoked paprika and drizzle with the remaining cilantro dressing. Squeeze the juice from the remaining lime half over the entire dish and serve.

continued

Smoked Paprika Chicken over Roasted Pepper–Corn Salad (continued)

Healthy Kitchen Hack: Don't throw out the water after the chicken is cooked! Remove the vegetables with a strainer and save the liquid for when you need chicken broth as an ingredient or want to make homemade soup like our Italian Wedding Soup with Meatballs (page 104). The broth will also keep in the freezer in a freezer-proof container for up to 6 months.

Per Serving: Calories: 319; Total Fat: 15g; Saturated Fat: 2g; Cholesterol: 83mg; Sodium: 347mg; Total Carbohydrates: 22g; Fiber: 5g; Protein: 28g

"This dish was a great mix of fresh flavors and colors! With the leftovers, I chopped up the chicken and mixed it with the corn salad for a cold lunch the next day."

—Ellen from Doylestown, PA

Moroccan Spice-Rubbed Chicken Thighs

Dairy-Free, Nut-Free, Gluten-Free, Egg-Free		Serves 4	Prep time: 10 minutes	Cook time: 15 minutes

½ teaspoon ground cumin

¼ teaspoon ground cinnamon

¼ teaspoon garlic powder

¼ teaspoon kosher or sea salt

¼ teaspoon black pepper

⅛ teaspoon ground allspice or ground ginger

4 (4-ounce) boneless, skinless chicken thighs

1 tablespoon extra-virgin olive oil

8 cups baby spinach

2 cups chopped fresh cilantro

After making this chicken, you may find yourself adding this aromatic cumin-and-cinnamon spice rub to many other foods like roasted vegetables, fish fillets, or grain bowls—it's that good. Triple or quadruple the spice blend amounts to keep on hand in your spice drawer or to give away as a gift. You can even add it to chili, stews, or canned soups to amp up the homemade flavor—and the antioxidant content, as these particular spices are rich sources of these disease-fighters.

In a small bowl, combine the cumin, cinnamon, garlic powder, salt, black pepper, and allspice. Rub the spice mixture over each chicken thigh.

In a large skillet over medium-high heat, heat the olive oil. Add the chicken and cook until just golden on both sides, or until the internal temperature of the chicken is 165°F on a meat thermometer, about 5 minutes on each side. Using a slotted spoon, remove the chicken to a plate, reserving the chicken drippings in the skillet.

Reduce the heat to medium. Add the spinach and cilantro to the skillet and cook, stirring constantly, until the spinach is wilted, 1 to 2 minutes. Top the spinach with the chicken and serve out of the skillet.

Healthy Kitchen Hack: Don't toss those pan drippings. The juices left in the pan after cooking lean meats in olive oil can be a gold mine, helpful for getting your family to enjoy more veggies. To help your pan juices help you, add any of the following to the pan after removing the meat or poultry and cook until just tender-crisp: hearty leafy greens, fresh herbs, carrots, broccoli, cabbage, snap peas, zucchini, shredded potatoes, and more.

Per Serving: Calories: 187; Total Fat: 9g; Saturated Fat: 2g; Cholesterol: 107mg; Sodium: 280mg; Total Carbohydrates: 3g; Fiber: 2g; Protein: 24g

Lemon-Oregano Chicken with Zucchini Noodles

| Nut-Free, Gluten-Free, Egg-Free | Serves 4 | Prep time: 15 minutes | Cook time: 15 minutes |

1 medium lemon

1 pound chicken tenders, cut into 1-inch pieces

3½ tablespoons extra-virgin olive oil, divided

1 tablespoon dried oregano

3 garlic cloves, minced

½ teaspoon kosher or sea salt, divided

½ teaspoon black pepper, divided

¼ teaspoon crushed red pepper

2 large or 3 small zucchini (14 to 16 ounces total)

3 tablespoons grated Parmesan or Pecorino Romano cheese

When you need to use up that zucchini in the summer, this dinner recipe with Greek-inspired flavors is your answer. You'll get a hefty serving of veggies and an appealing meal on the table in less than 30 minutes. Deanna likes to pair this dish with crusty whole-grain bread with Olive Oil–Yogurt Spread (page 42) for dipping.

Grate the lemon zest with a Microplane or citrus zester into a large bowl. Cut the lemon in half and squeeze all the juice into the bowl. Add the chicken, 2 tablespoons of the olive oil, the oregano, garlic, ¼ teaspoon of the salt, ¼ teaspoon of the black pepper, and the crushed red pepper. Using tongs or your hands, mix all the ingredients together until the chicken is well coated. Cover the bowl with a clean dish towel and set aside (for no more than 20 minutes).

While the chicken marinates, make the zucchini noodles using a spiralizer or a box grater. (See the Healthy Kitchen Hack on page 165 for more details on how to make zucchini noodles.) Add the noodles to a large bowl and toss with the remaining ¼ teaspoon salt and ¼ teaspoon black pepper. Set aside.

In a large skillet over medium heat, heat the remaining 1½ tablespoons olive oil. Add the chicken and cook, stirring occasionally with tongs, until it is no longer pink, 9 to 10 minutes.

Wash the tongs and then use them to add the zucchini noodles to the skillet with the chicken. Toss the noodles and the chicken together and cook, stirring occasionally with the tongs, until the zucchini has softened, 3 to 4 minutes. Sprinkle with the grated cheese and serve.

continued

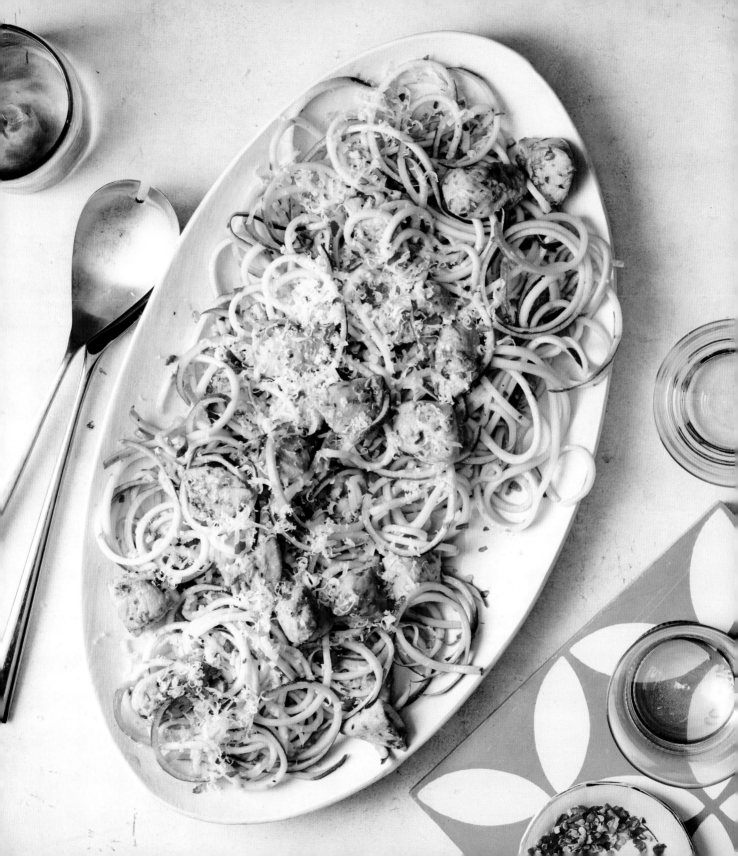

Healthy Kitchen Hack: For an even speedier dinner (less than 5 minutes of cooking time!), swap in canned chicken, canned tuna, or canned salmon for the chicken tenders. Mix the zucchini noodles with the olive oil and spices instead of the chicken tenders. Cook the noodles over medium heat for 3 to 4 minutes. Toss the canned fish or canned chicken with the zucchini noodles after you take them off the heat. Mix in the grated cheese and serve.

Per Serving: Calories: 293; Total Fat: 17g; Saturated Fat: 3g; Cholesterol: 86mg; Sodium: 372mg; Total Carbohydrates: 8g; Fiber: 2g; Protein: 29g

"This dish worked great for a light weeknight dinner. I LOVED the zoodles— they were excellent! They exceeded my expectations and would make a terrific lunch."

—Ellen from Havertown, PA

Saucy Sheet Pan Chicken with Sweet Potatoes

Dairy-Free, Nut-Free, Egg-Free	Serves 4	Prep time: 15 minutes	Cook time: 30 minutes

2 tablespoons tomato paste

1 tablespoon white wine vinegar or rice vinegar

1 tablespoon extra-virgin olive oil

1 tablespoon honey

1 teaspoon garlic powder

½ teaspoon fennel seeds or 1 teaspoon dried thyme

½ teaspoon plus ⅛ teaspoon kosher or sea salt, divided

1 medium red onion, cut into 8 wedges, divided

4 (6-ounce) bone-in, skin-on chicken thighs

3 small sweet potatoes (1 pound), unpeeled, scrubbed and cut into 1-inch cubes

1 tablespoon white whole-wheat flour

¼ cup white wine or low-sodium chicken broth

Serena was lucky enough to spend her honeymoon on the Greek island of Santorini. One day, she convinced her new husband to walk the very long, windy trail to the tip of the island. The views were spectacular and so were all the plants growing along the way, including wild fennel. Now the sweet, anise flavor of fennel seeds is one of Serena's favorite flavors. Here it's used to add a hint of sweetness to these mouth-watering marinated chicken thighs—a hands-down favorite of Serena's husband's (of twenty years!).

Preheat the oven to 425°F. Coat a large rimmed baking sheet with cooking spray.

To a blender, add ¼ cup water and the tomato paste, vinegar, olive oil, honey, garlic powder, fennel seeds, ½ teaspoon of the salt, and 1 of the onion wedges. Puree until smooth. Pour into a large bowl. Add the remaining onion wedges, the chicken thighs, and the sweet potato pieces. Using your hands or tongs, mix the tomato marinade around until all the chicken, sweet potatoes, and onions are coated. Cover with a plate and let marinate for 10 minutes on the counter (or up to 24 hours in the refrigerator).

Place the chicken thighs skin-side up on the prepared baking sheet and arrange the vegetables around the chicken so there is as much space between each piece as possible. Cook for 25 to 30 minutes or until the internal temperature of the chicken measures 165°F on a meat thermometer and the potatoes have softened. Using tongs, transfer the chicken and vegetables to a serving platter. Pour 1 cup boiling water over the baking sheet and, using a spatula, scrape up all the browned drippings and sticky bits on the pan. Carefully pour the drippings into a medium saucepan. Set aside.

continued

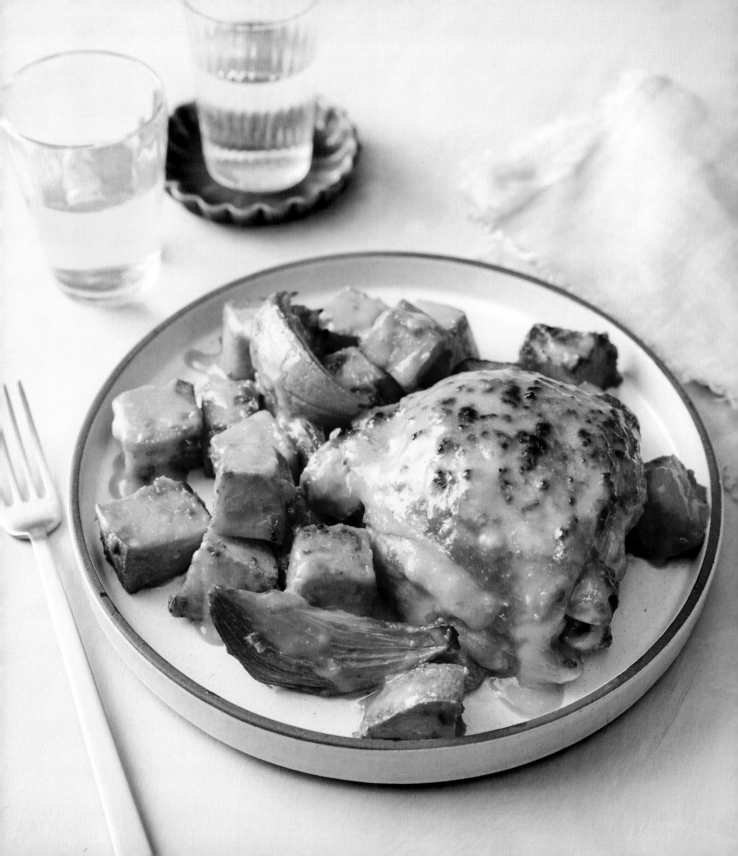

Saucy Sheet Pan Chicken with Sweet Potatoes (continued)

In a small bowl, combine the flour and wine. Whisk together until the flour dissolves. Pour into the saucepan with the drippings and whisk. Bring to a boil over medium-high heat, whisking occasionally. Cook, whisking frequently, until a slightly thick sauce forms, about 3 minutes. Remove from the heat and pour the sauce over the chicken and vegetables.

Healthy Kitchen Hack: To amp up the subtle fennel flavor in this recipe, substitute a bulb of fresh fennel for the red onion. Fennel has a slight anise flavor, similar to licorice, but more herbal. Cut the bulb into 8 wedges, reserving the fronds (the fennel's feathery leaves); use one wedge in the marinade and the remaining wedges as directed in the recipe. Chop the reserved fronds and use them to garnish the final dish.

Per Serving: Calories: 415; Total Fat: 15g; Saturated Fat: 3.5g; Cholesterol: 105mg; Sodium: 445mg; Total Carbohydrates: 35g; Fiber: 5g; Protein: 35g

Mediterranean Crispy Chicken and Potatoes

| Dairy-Free, Nut-Free, Egg-Free | Serves 4 | Prep time: 10 minutes | Cook time: 35 minutes |

1 tablespoon white whole-wheat flour

4 (6-ounce) bone-in, skin-on chicken thighs, trimmed

1 pound Yukon Gold potatoes (about 4 small), unpeeled, cut into ¾-inch cubes

4 garlic cloves, sliced

⅓ cup sliced green olives, ¼ cup liquid from the can or jar reserved

1 tablespoon dried oregano

½ teaspoon freshly ground black pepper

1 medium lemon, cut in half

The aroma of chicken frying in a cast iron skillet reminds Serena of her grandmother, who was known for her perfectly crunchy fried chicken at all the farms around her Montana ranch. This is our Mediterranean update of golden, crispy-skinned chicken with a bonus of fried potatoes on the side. Briny green olives and bright lemon flavors from the South of France add sunny flavors to the dish and slash the need for additional salt.

Preheat the oven to 425°F. Coat a large ovenproof or cast iron skillet with cooking spray.

In a small bowl, whisk together ½ cup water and the flour; set aside.

Pat the chicken dry with a paper towel and place skin-side down in the prepared skillet. Arrange the potatoes around the chicken so as many as possible are touching the cooking surface of the pan. (The potatoes may not all fit in the pan; place extra potatoes on top of the chicken.) Cover with a splatter screen if you have one. Cook over medium heat, turning the potatoes occasionally as they release from the pan. (The potatoes will release when a crisp side has formed. Without moving the chicken, keep rearranging the potatoes so that at least one side of the potatoes crisp.) Cook until the chicken skin releases from the pan and is golden and crispy, 14 to 16 minutes. Using tongs, turn the chicken skin-side up.

Place the skillet in the oven and bake for 11 to 13 minutes or until the internal temperature of the chicken measures 165°F on a meat thermometer and the potatoes have softened. Using a slotted spoon (to keep the juices in the skillet), transfer the chicken and potatoes to a plate. Set aside.

Place the skillet with the chicken juices back on the stovetop over medium heat. Add the garlic and cook, stirring frequently, for 1 minute. Add the flour-water mixture, the olive liquid, oregano, and black pepper and stir well. Cook, scraping up the charred bits on the bottom of the pan, until the pan sauce thickens, about 3 minutes.

Squeeze 1 tablespoon of lemon juice into the skillet. (Save any remaining lemon for another use.) Add the cooked chicken, potatoes, and olives and stir gently. Cook until heated through, 2 to 3 minutes, then serve from the skillet.

Healthy Kitchen Hack: Bone-in, skin-on chicken thighs are one of Serena's favorite poultry cuts to cook with; the bone and skin keep the meat flavorful and moist. The skin adds about 50 more calories and 1.5 g saturated fat over a skinless chicken thigh, but we've found an easy trimming can cut some of these calories and fat. Using kitchen shears, trim the skin so it is *only* covering the fleshy part of the thigh meat, not hanging over the edge of the thigh. If you decide to remove all the skin to save even more calories, do so after cooking, as the skin keeps the meat juicy.

Per Serving: Calories: 312; Total Fat: 11g; Saturated Fat: 3g; Cholesterol: 143mg; Sodium: 752mg; Total Carbohydrates: 27g; Fiber: 4g; Protein: 29g

"I loved the different flavor combo of lemons and olives along with chicken. It was nice to have a sunny Mediterranean dinner, as it's really snowy here. Next time I want to try it with chicken breasts!"

—Kristell from Billings, MT

White Wine–Roasted Chicken with Apples

| Dairy-Free, Nut-Free, Gluten-Free, Egg-Free | Serves 4 | Prep time: 10 minutes | Cook time: 25 minutes |

2 tablespoons extra-virgin olive oil

1 pound boneless, skinless chicken breasts, cut into 4 equal pieces total

3 medium apples, chopped

1 medium red onion, chopped

1 medium lemon, cut into wedges

1 tablespoon chopped fresh rosemary leaves

½ teaspoon kosher or sea salt

½ teaspoon black pepper

1½ cups dry white wine

We often think of citrus fruit and red wine grapes when it comes to Mediterranean cuisine because they tend to be warmer-climate plant species, but apples and white wine grapes are also actually native to the area. Deanna was amazed to see rolling hills of pear, cherry, and apple orchards along with white wine grape vineyards when visiting Israel. This white wine and apple chicken dish seems almost too simple to be as flavorful as it is—especially since you can have it ready in just a half hour with minimal prep.

Preheat the oven to 450°F degrees.

Pour the olive oil into an 11×13-inch metal baking pan. Add the chicken and flip a few times so the oil coats all the pieces. Add the apples, onion, lemon, rosemary, salt, and black pepper. Mix with your hands to ensure all the ingredients are equally distributed. Slowly pour the wine over the chicken. Cook, uncovered, for 22 to 25 minutes, until a meat thermometer inserted into the chicken registers 165°F and the wine has reduced down a bit.

Healthy Kitchen Hack: If you're feeding a few more people, opt for a 4- or 5-pound whole chicken using this same recipe. Cooking time will of course increase but the oven will be doing all the work. Roast for 45 to 60 minutes, until a meat thermometer inserted into the thickest part of the thigh (without touching the bone) registers 165°F.

Per Serving: Calories: 291; Total Fat: 10g; Saturated Fat: 2g; Cholesterol: 83mg; Sodium: 294mg; Total Carbohydrates: 23g; Fiber: 4g; Protein: 26g

Turkey Shawarma

Nut-Free, Egg-Free		Serves 6	Prep time: 10 minutes	Cook time: 20 minutes

1½ pounds turkey cutlets or breast, cut into 6 pieces

2 tablespoons extra-virgin olive oil, divided

1 teaspoon ground cumin, divided

½ teaspoon smoked paprika

½ teaspoon ground turmeric

¼ teaspoon kosher or sea salt

¼ teaspoon plus ⅛ teaspoon ground cinnamon, divided

¼ teaspoon black pepper

1 large red or sweet onion, thinly sliced

Olive Oil–Yogurt Spread (page 42)

1 cup chopped Spicy Sweet Quick Pickles (page 51)

¾ cup chopped tomatoes

6 (7- to 8-inch) whole-wheat pita breads, toasted

Move over, Thanksgiving! This aromatic recipe gives a flavor wake-up call to humdrum plain turkey breast. Shawarma is a Middle Eastern staple traditionally made with sliced seasoned beef or lamb, wrapped in pita and mixed with tantalizing condiments like smoky hummus, spicy pickles, relish-style tomatoes, and more. These days, you can find shawarma made with everything from goat to fish or, in this case, turkey. Deanna enjoys this version with a drizzle of tahini over top. Or try it with a schmear of our Smoky Baba Ghanoush Dip (page 49) in place of the yogurt spread used below.

Place each piece of turkey between two pieces of plastic wrap. Using a meat mallet, metal ladle, or a small frying pan, pound each piece down to a ¾-inch thickness. In a large glass bowl, add the turkey pieces, 1 tablespoon of the olive oil, ¾ teaspoon of the cumin, the smoked paprika, turmeric, the salt, ¼ teaspoon of the cinnamon, and the black pepper. Using tongs or your hands, mix and massage the marinade into the turkey pieces until they are completely coated. Set aside.

Into a small bowl, put the sliced onion, remaining ¼ teaspoon cumin, and remaining ⅛ teaspoon cinnamon. Stir to coat.

In a large skillet, heat 1 tablespoon of the olive oil over medium heat. Add the seasoned onions and cook, stirring occasionally, until the onions soften, about 10 minutes. Scrape the onions out of the pan into a bowl and set aside.

Return the skillet to the stove over medium heat (no need to wipe the pan clean) and add the turkey pieces. Cook, turning halfway through the cooking time, until a meat thermometer registers 165°F, 7 to 8 minutes. Cool for 5 minutes on a cutting board and then thinly slice.

continued

While the turkey cooks, make the Olive Oil–Yogurt Spread and set aside.

Divide the turkey among six serving plates. Top each with Olive Oil–Yogurt Spread, cooked onions, chopped pickles, and chopped tomatoes. Serve each with a side of toasted pita bread. If you prefer to serve this sandwich style, cut the pita in half, smear the yogurt spread inside the pita, and stuff with the remaining ingredients.

Healthy Kitchen Hack: Make this with seafood! Use 1½ pounds uncooked shrimp (peels and tails removed) instead of the turkey. Marinate with the same amount of oil and spices. Cook in a skillet over medium heat for about 5 minutes. Or use 1½ pounds white fish fillets, such as cod or tilapia, cut into 6 pieces. Cook for 8 to 10 minutes or until the fish just starts to flake.

Per Serving: Calories: 389; Total Fat: 10g; Saturated Fat: 2g; Cholesterol: 67mg; Sodium: 672mg; Total Carbohydrates: 41g; Fiber: 5g; Protein: 36g

Marinara Chicken-Lentil Bake

Dairy-Free, Nut-Free, Gluten-Free, Egg-Free	Serves 4	Prep time: 5 minutes	Cook time: 25 minutes

1 (26-ounce) jar low-sodium tomato pasta sauce or Easy Roasted Tomato Sauce (page 147)

1 cup dried brown lentils, rinsed

1½ cups chopped fresh parsley, divided

¼ teaspoon kosher or sea salt

¼ teaspoon black pepper

4 (4-ounce) boneless, skinless chicken thighs

This recipe is a bit of a revelation. Who knew you could cook lentils in the oven? (We didn't, until we tried it!) We do know, however, that we love lentils. They are rich in plant proteins, iron, and folate, and are super-affordable. They are also usually enjoyed even by bean-haters (Serena's youngest child is a case in point). This colorful dish couldn't be simpler and is a yummy way to introduce more lentils into your life.

Preheat the oven to 400°F.

In a large skillet, stir together 2½ cups water, the pasta sauce, and the lentils. Bring to a boil over high heat. Reduce the heat to medium and cook for 10 minutes. Stir in 1 cup of the parsley. Sprinkle the salt and black pepper over the chicken thighs and then nestle them into the warm sauce, making sure the chicken is covered.

Transfer the skillet to the oven and bake, uncovered, turning the skillet halfway to ensure even cooking, for 15 to 20 minutes or until the lentils have softened and the internal temperature of the chicken measures 165°F on a meat thermometer. Remove from the oven and mix in the remaining parsley.

Healthy Kitchen Hack: Don't have jarred tomato pasta sauce on hand? If you have a can of crushed tomatoes in your Mediterranean pantry (as we recommend stocking on page 11), you can whip up an easy substitute for jarred pasta sauce for any recipe, including this one. Mix together a 28-ounce can of crushed tomatoes, 1 tablespoon dried oregano, 1 tablespoon red wine vinegar, 1 teaspoon garlic powder, and ½ teaspoon black pepper. Heat in a small pot.

Per Serving: Calories: 352; Total Fat: 6g; Saturated Fat: 1g; Cholesterol: 107mg; Sodium: 427mg; Total Carbohydrates: 38g; Fiber: 8g; Protein: 36g

Sticky Lemon Chicken Drummies

Dairy-Free, Nut-Free, Gluten-Free, Egg-Free	Serves 4	Prep time: 10 minutes	Cook time: 25 minutes

8 chicken drumsticks with skin (about 2 pounds)

1 tablespoon cornstarch

2 medium lemons, cut in half

¼ cup honey

½ teaspoon garlic powder

½ teaspoon kosher or sea salt

¼ teaspoon black pepper

¼ teaspoon smoked paprika

Even if it's chilly outside, these bright, lemony drumsticks will fill your kitchen with Mediterranean sunshine. The spicy, sweet aromas will have everyone asking, "What's for dinner?"

Set one oven rack about 4 inches from the broiler. Preheat the oven to 500°F. Line a large rimmed baking sheet with aluminum foil. Place a wire rack on the baking sheet. Coat both with cooking spray. Arrange the chicken on the rack.

Into a medium saucepan, measure 2 tablespoons water and the cornstarch; whisk to combine. Squeeze ¼ cup of lemon juice into the pan. Add the honey, garlic powder, salt, black pepper, and smoked paprika and whisk to combine. Heat over medium heat until the mixture starts to boil, stirring often. Cook until just thickened, stirring constantly, 1 to 2 minutes. Remove from the heat and divide the glaze into two small bowls (reserve one for serving). Brush the chicken on all sides with glaze. Bake for 10 minutes. Remove the baking sheet from the oven. Turn on the broiler to high.

Using tongs, turn over each drumstick. Place under the broiler for 4 to 5 minutes until the drumsticks just begin to darken. Remove and turn with clean tongs. Broil for 2 to 3 minutes longer until the drumsticks start to turn dark brown and the internal temperature of the chicken measures 165°F on a meat thermometer. Serve with the reserved glaze.

Healthy Kitchen Hack: Use this glaze for chicken breasts, chicken thighs, pork chops, or lamb chops. It's spicy and sweet but with a fraction of the sugar of most bottled barbecue sauces. And since it's made with honey, it helps keep chicken moist while clinging to meat.

Per Serving: Calories: 309; Total Fat: 10g; Saturated Fat: 3g; Cholesterol: 110mg; Sodium: 254mg; Total Carbohydrates: 14g; Fiber: 0g; Protein: 39g

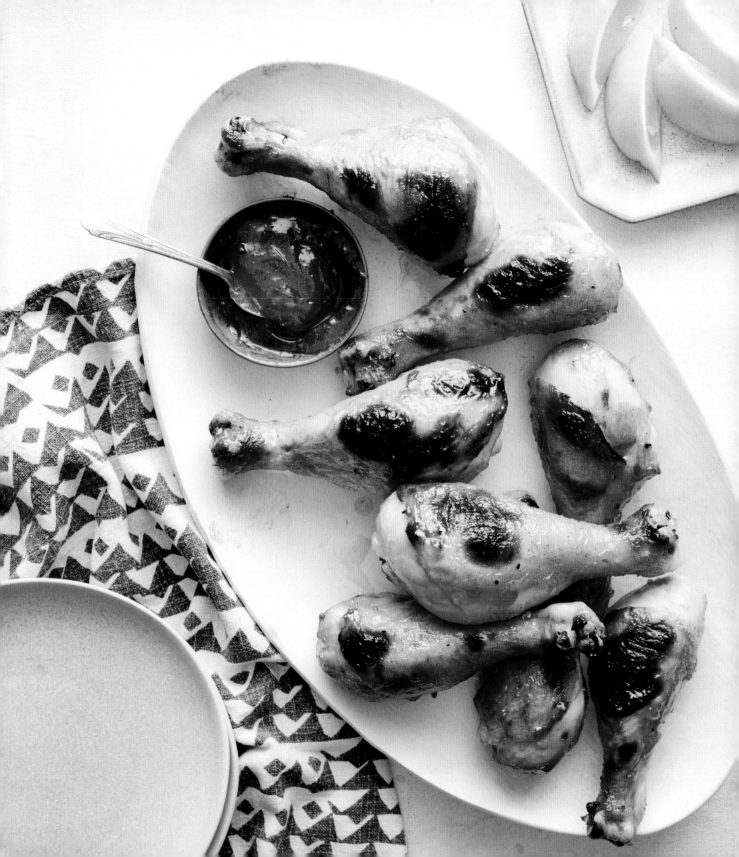

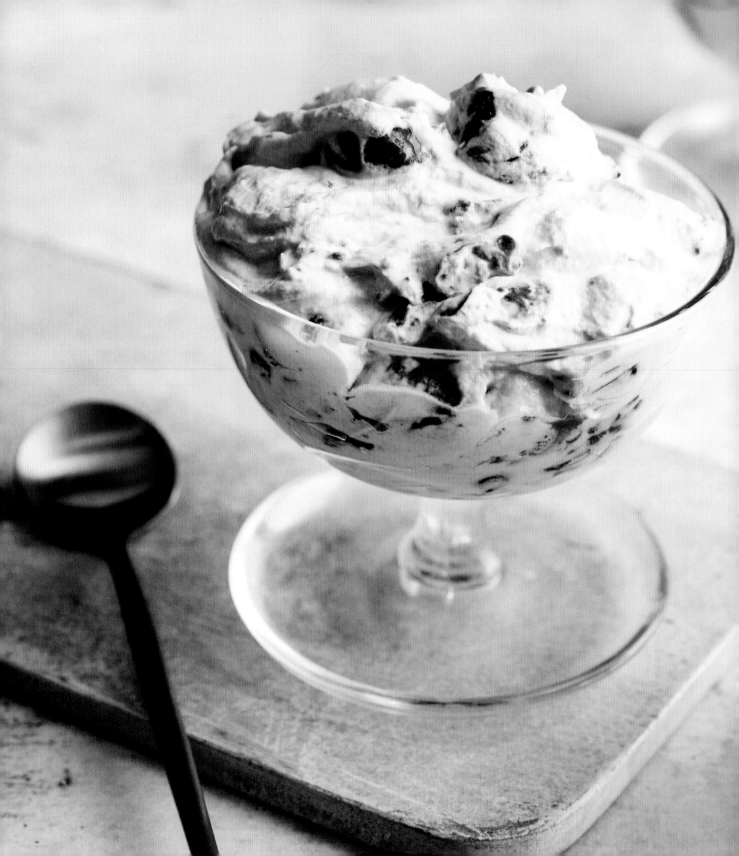

desserts

Frozen Mango Whip

Dairy-Free, Nut-Free, Gluten-Free, Egg-Free, Vegan	Serves 4	Prep time: 10 minutes

1 (16-ounce) package frozen mango

⅛ teaspoon plus a dash more of kosher or sea salt

1 medium lemon, cut in half

Smoked paprika (optional)

Dessert is not a typical part of the Mediterranean lifestyle—it's usually saved for special occasions. A more common way to end the meal is with a serving of fruit, and we can't wait for you try this whipped frozen mango that's super-creamy but also dairy free! Once you master this recipe, try other combinations like frozen grapes, frozen peaches mixed with mango, or frozen bananas with instant coffee granules.

Into a food processor or high-powered blender, put the frozen mango and ⅛ teaspoon of the salt. Process until the mango is very smooth and ice cream–like. (First, it will be tiny pebbles, but keep processing until smooth.) Cut the lemon in half and squeeze 2 teaspoons of the juice into the food processor. (Save any remaining lemon for another use.) Pulse two or three times until mixed.

Scoop the mango whip into serving bowls and, if desired, sprinkle with smoked paprika and additional salt.

Healthy Kitchen Hack: While frozen fruit is a bargain, canned fruit is even less expensive—so we tested this recipe using a 20-ounce can of pineapple chunks in 100 percent juice. Drain the pineapple and reserve the juice for another use. Place the pineapple chunks on a parchment paper–covered baking sheet and freeze for 2 hours. Blend following the directions above. Serve the pineapple whip with a sprinkle of ground ginger or black pepper, if desired.

Per Serving: Calories: 75; Total Fat: 0g; Saturated Fat: 0g; Cholesterol: 0mg; Sodium: 61mg; Total Carbohydrates: 19g; Fiber: 2g; Protein: 1g

Mini Tiramisu Bread Puddings

Nut-Free, Vegetarian		Serves 12	Prep time: 15 minutes	Cook time: 20 minutes

3 large eggs

⅓ cup sugar

2 tablespoons plus
1 teaspoon honey, divided

2¼ cups reduced-fat (2%)
milk, divided

1 tablespoon plus ¾ teaspoon
instant espresso granules,
divided

½ cup vanilla Greek yogurt

1 teaspoon vanilla extract

¼ teaspoon kosher or sea salt

7 cups cubed toasted Italian
bread

1 cup mascarpone cheese
(8 ounces)

1 tablespoon unsweetened
dark cocoa powder

This mash-up dessert reflects two of Deanna's favorite sweet treats: Italian coffee-flavored tiramisu and bread pudding. These individualized desserts are baked in a muffin tin for built-in portion control and a fun presentation. We use less sugar and replace the heavy cream with milk and yogurt to make the ending to your Mediterranean meal a bit lighter but just as satisfying.

Preheat the oven to 350°F. Coat a 12-cup muffin tin with cooking spray.

Into a large bowl, put the eggs, sugar, and 2 tablespoons of the honey. Whisk together well. Add 2 cups of the milk, 1 tablespoon of the espresso granules, the yogurt, vanilla, and salt. Whisk together well. Add the cubed bread and toss until all the pieces are soaked in the liquid. Let sit for 5 minutes or until most of the liquid is absorbed.

Divide the soaked bread into the prepared muffin tin cups. Bake for 18 to 20 minutes, until a toothpick inserted into the center comes out clean.

While the bread puddings cook, in a small bowl, add the mascarpone cheese, the remaining 1 teaspoon honey, and the remaining ¾ teaspoon espresso granules. Whisk together while slowly drizzling in the remaining ¼ cup milk.

Place each warm bread pudding on a small plate and drizzle with the mascarpone sauce. Sprinkle with the cocoa powder and serve.

Healthy Kitchen Hack: To make a mocha (aka coffee plus chocolate!) version of this recipe, swap in dark chocolate for the sugar. You can use dark chocolate chips or take a dark chocolate bar and chop it up into small bits.

Per Serving: Calories: 234; Total Fat: 11g; Saturated Fat: 6g; Cholesterol: 77mg; Sodium: 247mg; Total Carbohydrates: 26g; Fiber: 1g; Protein: 7g

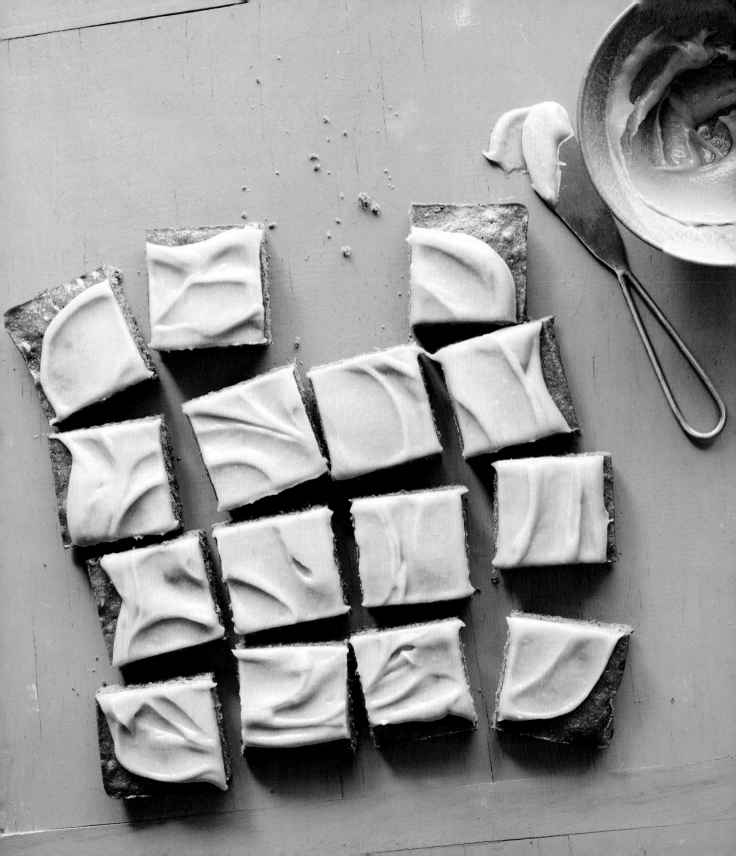

Tahini Brownies

Dairy-Free, Nut-Free, Vegetarian	Serves 16	Prep time: 10 minutes	Cook time: 20 minutes

⅔ cup white whole-wheat flour or whole-wheat pastry flour

⅓ cup unsweetened dark cocoa powder

¼ teaspoon baking powder

¼ teaspoon kosher or sea salt

¾ cup plus 2 tablespoons tahini, divided

½ cup sugar

⅓ cup plus 2 tablespoons honey, divided

2 large eggs

2 tablespoons extra-virgin olive oil

1 medium lemon, cut in half

1 teaspoon vanilla extract

Tahini is the special ingredient in these scrumptious, chocolatey brownies but it's up to you if you want to share the secret. Much like peanut butter in desserts, the nutty, earthy, and slightly sweet flavor of the sesame paste is a terrific match for dark chocolate. Along with adding more heart-healthy fats and fiber, we've reduced the total added sugar and fat content—even with the honey-tahini icing.

Preheat the oven to 350°F. Coat an 8- or 9-inch square metal baking pan with cooking spray.

In a large bowl, whisk together the flour, cocoa powder, baking powder, and salt. Set aside.

In another bowl, whisk together ½ cup of the tahini, the sugar, ⅓ cup of the honey, the eggs, olive oil, and vanilla. Pour into the dry ingredients. Mix together until a thick batter forms.

Pour the batter into the prepared pan and spread it out evenly to each corner. Bake for 16 to 18 minutes or until the edges are visibly baked through and the center is just set. Remove the pan from the oven, place on a wire rack, and cool for 15 minutes.

While the brownies bake, squeeze 1 tablespoon of lemon juice into a small bowl. (Save any remaining lemon for another use.) Add the remaining 6 tablespoons tahini, remaining 2 tablespoons honey, and 2 tablespoons water to small bowl. Whisk together until the icing is thick and smooth.

Once the brownies have cooled, spread on the icing over the top, then cut into 16 squares.

continued

Tahini Brownies (continued)

Healthy Kitchen Hack: While white whole-wheat flour is a staple in our pantries, Deanna also likes the lightness of whole-wheat pastry flour when it comes to baking sweet treats. In general, regular pastry flour is a lower-protein and lower-gluten flour that is milled to be lighter in texture than all-purpose flour. Whole-wheat pastry flour is just a touch denser and brings along some extra nutrients, but it is still very mild and can be a bit more palatable compared to other heavier whole-wheat flour options.

Per Serving: Calories: 159; Total Fat: 8g; Saturated Fat: 1g; Cholesterol: 23mg; Sodium: 43mg; Total Carbohydrates: 21g; Fiber: 2g; Protein: 4g

"These brownies have great texture and flavor. They would taste yummy even without the icing. My family loved them, and I will definitely make them again!"

—Rachel from St. Paul, MN

Cannoli Cups

Nut-Free, Gluten-Free, Egg-Free, Vegetarian	Serves 6	Prep time: 10 minutes

1 (15-ounce) container part-skim ricotta cheese

4 ounces mascarpone cheese

1 tablespoon honey

½ teaspoon vanilla extract

¼ teaspoon ground nutmeg

1 medium orange

⅓ cup mini chocolate chips

In Deanna's HIO (Humble Italian Opinion), the very best part of a cannoli is the silky-smooth, creamy ricotta filling. Years ago, her cousin brought a cannoli dip to her baby shower and it was a revelation to eat a cannoli this way—with the filling being the star of the show and the crispy pastry shells broken into pieces for dipping. Our portion-controlled variation features a few Mediterranean ingredients—mascarpone cheese, honey, and orange zest—and you can whip it up in minutes. If you miss the crunch of the shell, feel free to add some broken-up pieces of graham crackers.

In the bowl of a stand mixer or in a large bowl, add the ricotta, mascarpone, honey, vanilla, and nutmeg. Beat with the stand mixer paddle attachment or with electric beaters until very smooth, 1½ to 2 minutes.

Grate the peel of the orange with a Microplane or a citrus zester over the bowl. (Save any remaining orange for another use.) Add the chocolate chips and gently mix in with a rubber spatula. Divide among six ramekins or wine glasses and serve.

Healthy Kitchen Hack: During the fall, Deanna likes to add canned pumpkin puree to this dessert for a seasonal sweet treat. She usually mixes in 1 cup, but you can add whatever amount you have left over from the can. (Why do so many pumpkin recipes not call for the entire can?) It's up to you whether you want to jump on the pumpkin spice bandwagon and also mix in ½ teaspoon ground cinnamon, ¼ teaspoon ground ginger, and ¼ teaspoon ground allspice or ground cloves.

Per Serving: Calories: 253; Total Fat: 17g; Saturated Fat: 11g; Cholesterol: 49mg; Sodium: 77mg; Total Carbohydrates: 15g; Fiber: 1g; Protein: 9g

Blueberry-Peach Crostata

Dairy-Free, Nut-Free, Egg-Free, Vegetarian	Serves 8	Prep time: 15 minutes	Cook time: 30 minutes

1 refrigerated pie crust for a 9-inch pie

1 medium lemon, cut in half

2 cups frozen sliced peaches or fresh unpeeled sliced peaches (about 12 ounces)

1½ cups frozen or fresh blueberries (about 6 ounces)

3 tablespoons plus ½ teaspoon honey, divided

1½ tablespoons white whole-wheat flour

¼ teaspoon kosher or sea salt

"I've made a lot of pies in my life, but this tart was even easier. And I like that I can use different combos of whatever fruit I have!"

—Janet from Huntley, MT

We find making pie frustrating. Getting the dough just right, transferring it to a pie plate, and hoping it doesn't shrink upon baking are just a few reasons we rarely make a traditional pie from scratch. Our solution? Make a fruit crostata, which is an Italian free-form pie—in other words, it doesn't have to look perfect! Some of our favorite Mediterranean fruit combinations for the filling include blackberries with apples, cherries with plums, and figs with oranges. And despite its simple assembly, this irresistible rustic pie always impresses guests.

Preheat the oven to 400°F. Line a large rimmed baking sheet with parchment paper. Unroll the pie crust on the parchment paper.

Squeeze 3 tablespoons of lemon juice into a medium saucepan. (Save any remaining lemon for another use.) Stir in the peaches, blueberries, 3 tablespoons of the honey, the flour, and the salt. Heat over medium-high heat until boiling, stirring often, until the liquid is thick and the fruit is tender, 6 to 8 minutes.

Using a large spoon, carefully pile the fruit filling in the center of the pie crust to within 2 inches of the edge. Fold the edges of the dough up and over the fruit, leaving the fruit in the center exposed in a 7- to 8-inch-wide circle. Press to seal the folded crust seams. Drizzle the remaining ½ teaspoon honey over the crust.

Bake for 25 to 30 minutes until the crust is golden brown and the fruit is bubbling. Let the crostata cool for at least 15 minutes on a wire rack before slicing.

Healthy Kitchen Hack: Even if you perfectly seal the edges of your crostata, fruit juice will still likely bubble out onto the parchment paper during baking. After the crostata comes out of the oven, carefully scoop up those juices and drizzle them back over the fruit filling. Once the crostata has cooled, slide a spatula under it to move it to a serving plate or cutting board.

Per Serving: Calories: 161; Total Fat: 6g; Saturated Fat: 3g; Cholesterol: 5mg; Sodium: 191mg; Total Carbohydrates: 28g; Fiber: 1g; Protein: 2g

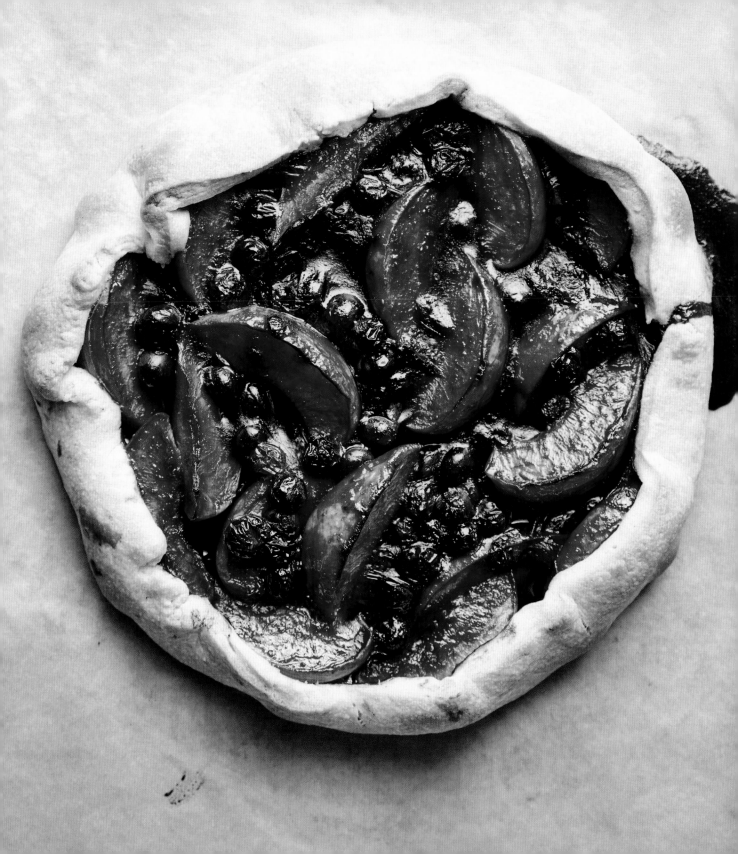

Honey-Panzanella Fruit Bowl

| Dairy-Free, Nut-Free, Vegetarian | Serves 8 | Prep time: 15 minutes | Cook time: 10 minutes |

6 cups 1-inch cubes challah bread (about 8 ounces)

2 tablespoons extra-virgin olive oil

1 large orange

7 cups chopped fruit (like cherries, apricots, peaches, apples, grapes, figs, and pomegranate seeds)

1 tablespoon honey

¾ teaspoon vanilla extract

¼ teaspoon kosher or sea salt

¼ cup fresh mint leaves, torn

Here we take the concept of panzanella—an Italian tomato-bread salad—and change it to a sweet ending by using challah bread and fruit. Vanilla extract is the aromatic secret ingredient, which makes it smell and taste like dessert—we now routinely add it to all our fruit cup recipes.

Preheat the oven to 400°F.

In a large shallow serving bowl, toss the cubed bread with the olive oil. Spread the cubes out evenly onto a large rimmed baking sheet. Bake, stirring once, for 6 to 8 minutes, until the bread cubes are toasted. Remove from the oven and set aside.

Grate the orange zest with a Microplane or citrus zester into the same large serving bowl. Cut the orange in half and squeeze all of the juice into the bowl. Add the chopped fruit, honey, vanilla, and salt. Using your hands, toss all the ingredients together. Let sit for at least 5 minutes.

Right before serving, add the toasted bread cubes and gently combine. Sprinkle with the torn mint and serve.

Healthy Kitchen Hack: You can also make this dessert using frozen or canned fruit. For frozen fruit, let it come to room temperature on your countertop and then drain. If using canned fruit, either drain it well or replace the orange juice with ½ cup of the canned fruit juice.

Per Serving: Calories: 227; Total Fat: 6g; Saturated Fat: 1g; Cholesterol: 6mg; Sodium: 232mg; Total Carbohydrates: 43g; Fiber: 3g; Protein: 4g

Mini Pomegranate-Apple Crisps

Gluten-Free, Egg-Free, Vegetarian	Serves 6	Prep time: 10 minutes	Cook time: 25 minutes

3 medium apples, chopped

1 cup pomegranate seeds

½ cup unsweetened applesauce

3 tablespoons honey, divided

½ teaspoon ground cinnamon

½ teaspoon vanilla extract

¼ teaspoon kosher or sea salt

½ cup gluten-free rolled oats

½ cup plus 2 tablespoons vanilla Greek yogurt, divided

⅓ cup Cinnamon-Fig Granola (page 23) or another granola

2 tablespoons ground flaxseed

1 tablespoon extra-virgin olive oil

"The vanilla and cinnamon really bring out the flavor in these! Delicious with vanilla ice cream."

—Olivia from Plymouth, MI

One of Deanna's many thrilling food takeaways from her Israel trip was the sheer abundance of ruby-red pomegranates. On display in open-air markets, growing in parking lots, and symbolized in works of art, this gorgeous fruit has been intertwined in Middle Eastern cultures for thousands of years. Here in the Northern Hemisphere, look for the whole fruit and packages of the seeds (called arils) from October through January. Just don't ask your grocer if they sell "seedless pomegranates" (like Deanna's friend innocently did after a coworker set her up!).

Preheat the oven to 375°F. Coat six 6-ounce ramekins with cooking spray.

Into a large microwave-safe bowl, put the apples and 2 tablespoons water. Microwave on high for 3 minutes (to jump-start cooking the apples).

To the bowl of heated apples, add the pomegranate seeds, applesauce, 2 tablespoons of the honey, the cinnamon, vanilla, and salt. Mix well and then divide evenly among the prepared ramekins.

In the same bowl, add the remaining 1 tablespoon honey, the oats, ¼ cup of the yogurt, the granola, flaxseed, and olive oil. Mix well and divide the topping evenly over the mixed fruit.

Place the ramekins on a large rimmed baking sheet and bake for 18 to 20 minutes, until the topping is golden brown and the fruit is bubbling. Remove from the oven and transfer the ramekins to a wire rack. Cool for 5 to 10 minutes. Top the crisps with the remaining 6 tablespoons yogurt before serving.

Healthy Kitchen Hack: To serve this family style, add the fruit filling to a 9×9-inch baking pan coated with cooking spray. Spread the crisp topping over the fruit and bake in a preheated 375°F oven for 25 to 30 minutes.

Per Serving: Calories: 227; Total Fat: 6g; Saturated Fat: 1g; Cholesterol: 1mg; Sodium: 103mg; Total Carbohydrates: 42g; Fiber: 6g; Protein: 4g

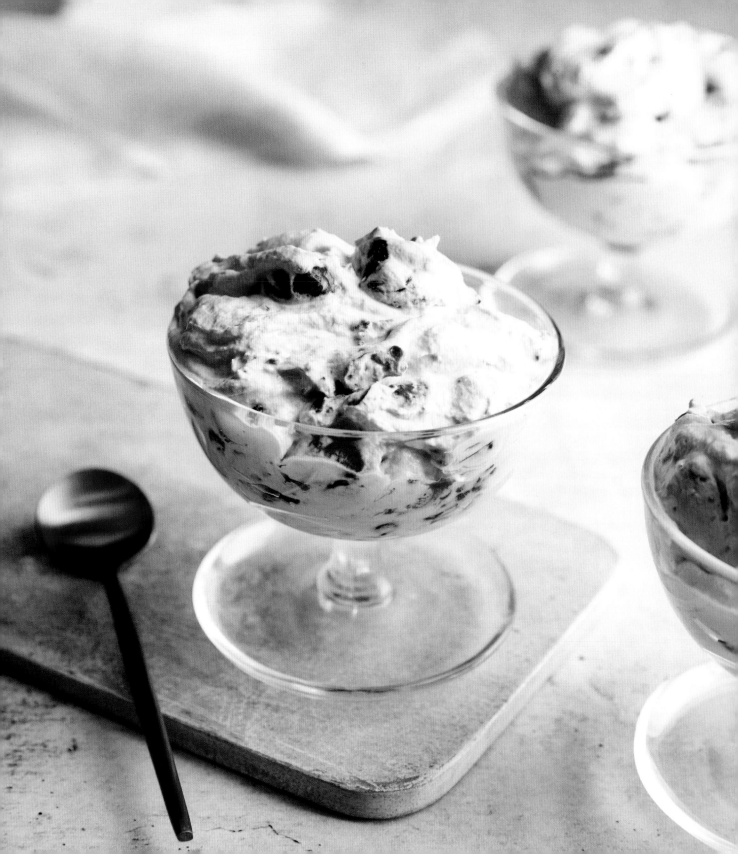

Cherry Cloud Dessert

Gluten-Free, Egg-Free, Vegetarian	Serves 6	Prep time: 25 minutes (includes chill time)	Cook time: 10 minutes

2 cups frozen sweet or tart cherries (about 9 ounces, divided)

1 cup plain 2% Greek yogurt (8 ounces)

1 medium lemon, cut in half

3 tablespoons honey, divided

1 tablespoon cornstarch

⅔ cup heavy (whipping) cream (6 ounces)

¼ teaspoon almond extract

Mint leaves, for serving (optional)

If there's one dessert technique you need in your culinary bag of tricks, it's making homemade whipped cream. Adding billowy clouds of whipped cream can turn desserts from decent to grand, and also make a serving of plain fruit into something special. Homemade whipped cream is the base to this wow-factor, cold dessert—ready in only 30 minutes, thanks to our hack of chilling the ingredients while you assemble the dessert.

Place the cherries on the counter to thaw slightly, about 5 minutes.

Place a large glass bowl and the metal beaters from your electric mixer in the refrigerator to chill.

Put the yogurt in a medium glass bowl and also place in the refrigerator to chill.

On a cutting board, chop 1 cup of the icy cherries. Squeeze 1 tablespoon of lemon juice into a microwave-safe medium bowl. (Save any remaining lemon for another use.) Add 2 tablespoons of the honey and the cornstarch and whisk together. Add the chopped cherries and stir well. Microwave the cherry mixture on high for 3 minutes; stir and microwave for an additional 2 to 4 minutes, until the mixture is thick and bubbling, stopping to stir after each minute of microwaving. Stir in the remaining 1 cup whole icy cherries.

Remove the bowl of yogurt from the refrigerator and fold in the warm cherry mixture. Place the bowl back into the refrigerator.

Remove the chilled empty large bowl and beaters from the refrigerator. Assemble your electric mixer with the chilled beaters. Pour the cream, remaining 1 tablespoon honey, and the almond extract into the chilled bowl. Beat until soft peaks form, 1 to 3 minutes, depending on the freshness of your cream.

continued

Cherry Cloud Dessert (continued)

Take the chilled yogurt mixture out of the refrigerator. Gently fold it into the whipped cream using a rubber spatula by lifting and turning the mixture to prevent the cream from deflating. Chill for at least 15 minutes but no longer than 3 hours before serving.

To serve, spoon the chilled dessert into four glasses or dessert dishes. Top with a few mint leaves, if desired.

Healthy Kitchen Hack: Make a thickened fruit sauce using the microwave technique you learned here. In a microwave-safe bowl, mix together 2 tablespoons honey, 1 tablespoon lemon juice, 1 tablespoon cornstarch, and 1 cup chopped fresh or frozen fruit such as peaches, plums, oranges, lemons, pears, apples, mangoes, blueberries, or any berry. The time to thicken the fruit will vary depending on the fruit, so stop and stir after each minute of microwaving to check the thickening.

Per Serving: Calories: 170; Total Fat: 11g; Saturated Fat: 7g; Cholesterol: 35mg; Sodium: 10mg; Total Carbohydrates: 18g; Fiber: 1g; Protein: 2g

Impossibly Good Lemon Bars

Vegetarian	Serves 12	Prep time: 15 minutes	Cook time: 30 minutes

1 cup white whole-wheat flour

¼ cup finely chopped pecans

¼ cup cornstarch, divided

½ teaspoon kosher or sea salt, divided

½ cup plus 2 tablespoons powdered sugar, divided

2 tablespoons extra-virgin olive oil

¼ cup plain 2% Greek yogurt (2 ounces)

3 medium lemons

¼ cup honey

3 large eggs

1 large egg yolk

At one point during the many rounds of this recipe's creation, Serena thought it might be "impossible" to pull off a Mediterranean update to old-fashioned lemon bars made with butter and sugar. But all of our taste testers agreed that her final version was a scrumptious success that uses pecans, olive oil, and Greek yogurt in the shortbread-like crust and honey to sweeten the tart lemon filling. If you are a lemon lover, this is a must-bake recipe—after all, it is the most tested one in the book!

Preheat the oven to 350°F. Coat a 9-inch square baking pan with cooking spray.

In a large bowl, combine the flour, pecans, 3 tablespoons of the cornstarch, and ¼ teaspoon of the salt.

Into a medium bowl, measure ½ cup of the powdered sugar, the olive oil, and the yogurt. Whisk together and scrape into the flour mixture. Combine with a fork or your hands. (The mixture should be dry and crumbly.)

Add the crust to the prepared pan. Using a rubber spatula or your hands, press until it has flattened and spread to reach the pan corners. Bake for 15 to 18 minutes, until firm in the center and the edges are just starting to turn golden. Remove the crust from the oven.

While the crust cooks, crack the eggs and egg yolk into a small bowl. Whisk until beaten and set aside.

Grate the zest of 1 lemon with a Microplane or citrus zester into a medium saucepan. Cut all 3 lemons in half and squeeze ½ cup of the juice into the pan. (Save any remaining lemon for another use.) Add the remaining 1 tablespoon cornstarch, the honey, and remaining ¼ teaspoon salt to the pan and whisk together. Cook over medium heat, whisking often to remove any lumps. Once the mixture bubbles, cook, stirring constantly, until the mixture thickens, about 1 minute. Reduce the heat to medium-low.

continued

In a steady slow stream, while whisking constantly, pour about 1 tablespoon of the hot mixture from the pan into the bowl with the eggs. Then slowly pour the egg mixture back into the saucepan, whisking constantly. Cook until the mixture begins to thicken, 4 to 5 minutes.

Carefully pour the hot lemon mixture over the baked crust. With oven mitts, hold the sides of the pan and tilt until the mixture is spread evenly. Return to the oven and bake for 5 to 7 more minutes, until the filling in the center is just dry. Remove from the oven and set on a wire rack. Let cool completely, then sprinkle with the remaining 2 tablespoons powdered sugar. Cut into 12 pieces and serve.

Healthy Kitchen Hack: As noted above, it can be pretty tricky to take a traditional baked-good recipe and convert it to include Mediterranean staples, as each ingredient is unique in its baking qualities. But start with the following conversions and then have fun tweaking it to get it "right":

1 cup butter = ½ cup olive oil plus ¼ cup plain 2% Greek yogurt
1 cup sugar = ½ cup plus 2 tablespoons honey and decrease the amount of liquid in the recipe by ¼ cup

Per Serving: Calories: 155, Total Fat: 6g; Saturated Fat: 1g; Cholesterol: 62mg; Sodium: 101mg; Total Carbohydrates: 24g; Fiber: 1g; Protein: 4g

"I'm not a big dessert person, but these were really good. I especially liked how the topping is really lemony and tart, but also sweet. Plus, lemons are my favorite fruit."

—David from Edwardsville, IL

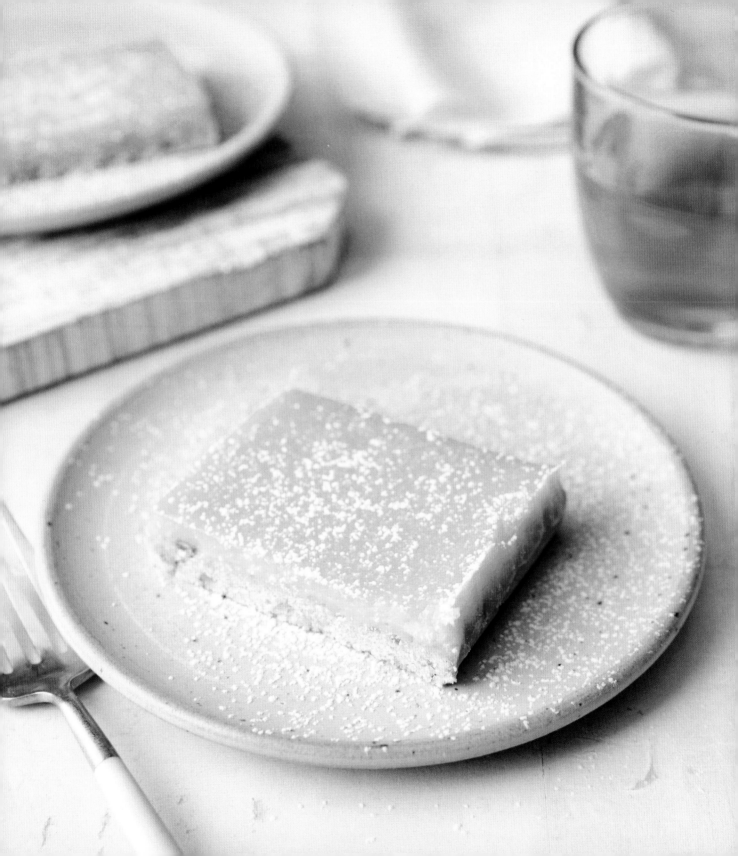

Appendix: Five-Day Meal Plans

	Gluten-Free	Vegetarian	Seafood 2x week	Meatless Monday
MONDAY				
Breakfast	Peanut Butter–Apricot Breakfast Oat Bars (made with gluten-free oats on the weekend)	Peanut Butter–Apricot Breakfast Oat Bars (made on the weekend)	Peanut Butter–Apricot Breakfast Oat Bars (made on the weekend)	Peanut Butter–Apricot Breakfast Oat Bars (made on the weekend)
Lunch	Kale Caesar Salad with Chickpeas (made with gluten-free bread for croutons), plain Greek yogurt with honey, fruit, and nuts	Kale Caesar Salad with Chickpeas, plain Greek yogurt with honey, fruit, and nuts	Kale Caesar Salad with Chickpeas, plain Greek yogurt with honey, fruit, and nuts	Kale Caesar Salad with Chickpeas, plain Greek yogurt with honey, fruit, and nuts
Snack	Hummus (from Smoky Baba Ghanoush Healthy Kitchen Hack) with raw veggies	Hummus (from Smoky Baba Ghanoush Healthy Kitchen Hack) with raw veggies	Hummus (from Smoky Baba Ghanoush Healthy Kitchen Hack) with raw veggies	Hummus (from Smoky Baba Ghanoush Healthy Kitchen Hack) with raw veggies
Dinner	Monday Minestrone Soup (made with gluten-free pasta on the weekend), chopped fruit salad	Monday Minestrone Soup (made on the weekend), chopped fruit salad	Monday Minestrone Soup (made on the weekend), chopped fruit salad	Monday Minestrone Soup (made on the weekend), chopped fruit salad
Dessert	Blackberry-Almond Energy Bites (made with gluten-free oats)	Blackberry-Almond Energy Bites	Blackberry-Almond Energy Bites	Blackberry-Almond Energy Bites
TUESDAY				
Breakfast	Leftover Peanut Butter–Apricot Breakfast Oat Bars (made with gluten-free oats)	Leftover Peanut Butter–Apricot Breakfast Oat Bars	Leftover Peanut Butter–Apricot Breakfast Oat Bars	Leftover Peanut Butter–Apricot Breakfast Oat Bars
Lunch	Leftover Monday Minestrone Soup, gluten-free crackers	Leftover Monday Minestrone Soup, whole-grain crackers	Leftover Monday Minestrone Soup, whole-grain crackers	Leftover Monday Minestrone Soup, whole-grain crackers
Snack	Blackberry-Almond Energy Bites (made with gluten-free oats)	Blackberry-Almond Energy Bites	Blackberry-Almond Energy Bites	Blackberry-Almond Energy Bites
Dinner	Lemon-Oregano Chicken with Zucchini Noodles, quinoa mixed with Olive Oil-Yogurt Spread	Sun-Dried Tomato Veggie Burgers, Herb Salad with Citrus-Date Dressing	Baked Salmon with Creamy Cilantro Sauce and Orange, Celery, and Olive Tabbouleh	Pepper-and-Sausage Skillet Supper (make extra Roasted Red Peppers), Arugula with Apricot Balsamic Dressing
Dessert	Frozen Mango Whip	Frozen Mango Whip	Frozen Mango Whip	Frozen Mango Whip
WEDNESDAY				
Breakfast	Tomato-Basil Frittata	Tomato-Basil Frittata	Tomato-Basil Frittata	Tomato-Basil Frittata
Lunch	Leftover Lemon-Oregano Chicken with Zucchini Noodles, leftover quinoa mixed with Olive Oil-Yogurt Spread	Leftover Sun-Dried Tomato Veggie Burgers, leftover Herb Salad with Citrus-Date Dressing	Leftover Baked Salmon with Creamy Cilantro Sauce (in a sandwich roll) and leftover Orange, Celery, and Olive Tabbouleh	Leftover Pepper-and-Sausage Skillet Supper, leftover Arugula with Apricot Balsamic Dressing
Snack	Grilled Watermelon Salad	Grilled Watermelon Salad	Grilled Watermelon Salad	Grilled Watermelon Salad

	Gluten-Free	Vegetarian	Seafood 2x week	Meatless Monday
Dinner	Loaded Mini Burgers on Grilled Sweet Potatoes, green salad	Oven-Baked Spinach-Feta Gnocchi, carrot and celery sticks	Oven-Baked Spinach-Feta Gnocchi, carrot and celery sticks	Roasted red pepper and tomato soup (from Easy Roasted Tomato Sauce Healthy Kitchen Hack), whole-grain bread, green salad
Dessert	A few pieces of dark chocolate	A few pieces of dark chocolate	A few pieces of dark chocolate	A few pieces of dark chocolate
THURSDAY				
Breakfast	Leftover Tomato-Basil Frittata	Leftover Tomato-Basil Frittata	Leftover Tomato-Basil Frittata	Leftover Tomato-Basil Frittata
Lunch	Leftover Loaded Mini Burgers on Grilled Sweet Potatoes	Leftover Oven-Baked Spinach-Feta Gnocchi, mini sweet peppers	Leftover Oven-Baked Spinach-Feta Gnocchi, mini sweet peppers	Leftover Roasted red pepper and tomato soup (from Easy Roasted Tomato Sauce Healthy Kitchen Hack), whole-grain crackers
Snack	Roasted grapes (from Roasted Grapes Cheese Plate), Honey-Roasted Pecans with Thyme	Roasted grapes (from Roasted Grapes Cheese Plate), Honey-Roasted Pecans with Thyme	Roasted grapes (from Roasted Grapes Cheese Plate), Honey-Roasted Pecans with Thyme	Roasted grapes (from Roasted Grapes Cheese Plate), Honey-Roasted Pecans with Thyme
Dinner	Roasted red pepper and tomato soup (from Easy Roasted Tomato Sauce Healthy Kitchen Hack), gluten-free crackers, green salad	Spaghetti Squash Noodles with Chickpea "Meatballs" (make extra "meatballs" for soup the next day), green salad	Skillet Shrimp with Tomatoes and Feta with whole-wheat pita bread, green salad	Greek Sloppy Yos (make extra meat-bean filling), Shredded Beet-and-Apple Slaw
Dessert	Fresh fruit	Fresh fruit	Fresh fruit	Fresh fruit
FRIDAY				
Breakfast	Apple-Walnut Ricotta Toast (on gluten-free bread)	Apple-Walnut Ricotta Toast	Apple-Walnut Ricotta Toast	Apple-Walnut Ricotta Toast
Lunch	Leftover roasted red pepper and tomato soup (from Easy Roasted Tomato Sauce Healthy Kitchen Hack), gluten-free crackers	Leftover roasted grapes paired with cheese, crackers, fruit, and veggies	Leftover Skillet Shrimp with Tomatoes and Feta, whole-wheat pita bread, fruit	Baked potatoes topped with Greek Sloppy Yos meat-bean filling, leftover Shredded Beet-and-Apple Slaw
Snack	Olive Oil-Yogurt Spread with raw veggies	Olive Oil-Yogurt Spread with raw veggies	Olive Oil-Yogurt Spread with raw veggies	Olive Oil-Yogurt Spread with raw veggies
Dinner	Leftover roasted grapes paired with cheese, smoked salmon, gluten-free crackers, fruit, and veggies for a dinner-size cheese board	Italian Wedding Soup with leftover Chickpea "Meatballs," whole-grain bread	Leftover roasted grapes paired with cheese, smoked salmon, crackers, fruit, and veggies for dinner-size cheese board	Leftover roasted grapes paired with cheese, smoked salmon, crackers, fruit, and veggies for dinner-size cheese board
Dessert	Mini Pomegranate-Apple Crisps (made with gluten-free oats and gluten-free granola)	Mini Pomegranate-Apple Crisps	Mini Pomegranate-Apple Crisps	Mini Pomegranate-Apple Crisps

Index

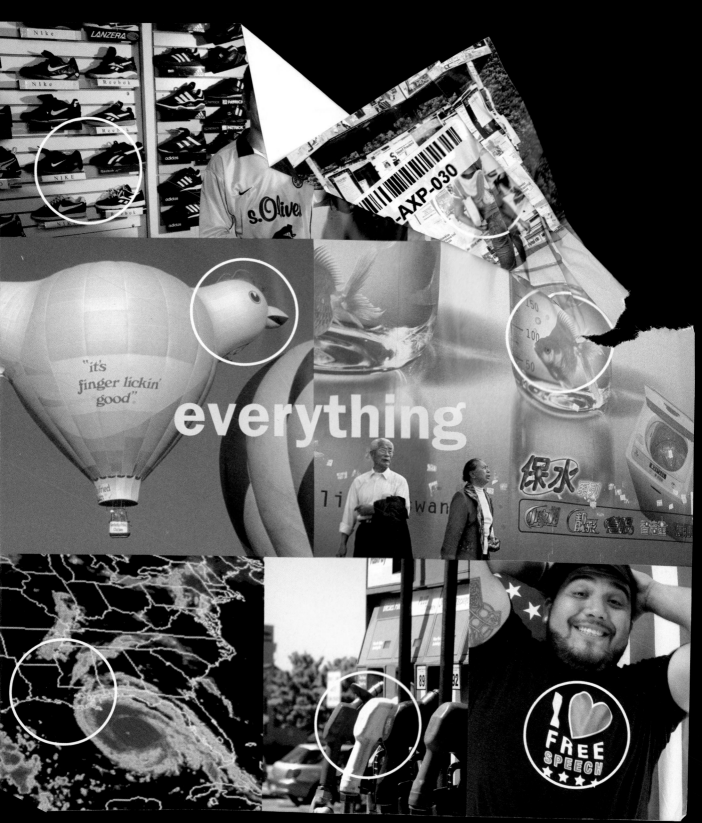